I0197699

COUNT ME IN

Large Group Activities that Work

by Mark Collard

Illustrations by Michelle Dybing

Copyright © 2008 by:

Project Adventure, Inc.
701 Cabot Street
Beverly MA 01915 USA
1 (978) 524-4500

Challenge by Choice and Full Value
Contract are registered service marks of
Project Adventure Inc. and may not be
used without the written permission of
Project Adventure Inc.

ISBN 978-0-934387-30-9

First printed in 2008
Printed in Australia 2015, 2018, 2021

10 9 8 7 6 5 4 3 2 1

Illustrations by Michelle Dybing

Book design and production by:
SYP Design & Production, Inc.
www.sypdesign.com

playmeo

Visit **playmeo.com/activities** to view 100s of fun group games &
activities, many of which are featured in this book. Get step-by-step
instructions, video tutorials, leadership tips & so much more.

Acknowledgements

I wish to thank the many thousands of participants who have willingly accepted the invitation to play in the countless programs I have delivered since the early eighties. The gems contained within these pages shine ever more brightly because you obliged me as I honed my facilitation skills and, as a result, the ability to positively impact large groups of people.

More specifically, I express enormous gratitude to a smaller group of people who have given me the space to play; namely the international Project Adventure team including: Rufus Collinson, Suze Collinson, Daryl Essensa, Tara Flippo, Ryan McCormick, Jane Panicucci, Dick Prouty and Alison Rheingold. Special mentions to Rodger Popkin and the whole Blue Star Camps family, for inviting me to share my love of summer camp programming in the USA for eight summers. I also say special thank yous to Peter Byrne, Don MacDowall, Pam Wood and my family, simply because you motivate me to laugh and have fun, and lots of it.

And finally, I reserve my deepest acknowledgement for two of the most extraordinary people in the world who have radically influenced the kind of person I am today – my most gorgeous wife Gilly, who inspires me no-end to be a better person everyday; and Karl Rohnke, who invited my initial foray into the world of adventure education.

Humbly, I thank you.

Contents

Introduction

A Formula for Success

If you want to run a successful program, take my advice – never work with young children. Nor should you think of working with animals – they too can be distracting! Oh, and if you really want a formula for success, never, ever, work with large groups!

Huh? Well, this is what I was actually told by some of my peers, way back when I started treading the metaphoric adventure programming boards for the first time. While I think the 'advice' was offered in good humour, it no doubt continues to reflect the cogitations of more than a few program providers out there today. Maybe even you?

Large groups are really like any other group – really! Except – and you don't have to be a rocket scientist to work this one out – they are much bigger.

Bigger, in terms of scariness, perhaps.

Bigger, because in the face of a gazillion pairs of eyes, they are more likely to provoke Anxiety.

Bigger, because they can generate a lot more fun, non-stop energy, and likely to have you asking for more? an emphatic YES!

I have loved working with large groups for all of these 'bigger' reasons; and believe me, I have experienced them all. Babies, young children, older adults, the lot. Although, sadly, no animals – unless you want to include a curious roaming dog or two, and there was once this emu who stole my fleece-balls! But, that's another story.

What Is a Large Group?

So, how big is a 'large' group you might ask? Well, I could numerate, but let me conduct a quick test first. In my experience, you are working with a large group if:

(a) You ran out of sticky labels for name-tags within two minutes of people arriving;

(b) You ask your group to stand in a circle, and as you see it form, you say to yourself "Whoooaaa...., there really ARE a lot of people here;"

(c) You consider yourself good with names, but you've decided to skip the name-game today;

(d) The very thought of standing in front of this audience makes you start to perspire; or

(e) You have found yourself doing all of the above, often at the same time.

If you have nodded or grinned to at least one of these scenarios, consider yourself at work with a 'large' group – no matter what size. This book is dedicated to you, as well as to anyone who simply enjoys the energy and sheer craziness that only a large group can add to a program. But for practical purposes, I'm talking numbers in excess of 30 to 50 people safe enough to be called a 'large' group.

Much like a bag full of 'no prop' activities that you can whip out of your back-pocket at a moment's notice, you can never have enough activity ideas for large groups. That's what this book is all about. It is full of sure-fire, high-energy, interactive, leave-them-wanting-for-more activities.

Every activity is coupled with at least one variation, and often two or more. So, really, you're picking up a vast treasure chest of programming ideas, perfect for any group of people, especially if there are a lot of them.

Have fun! And remember, look out for crying babies and the occasional roving emu!

About Project Adventure

It is more than just the name of an organisation. Project Adventure is an approach to working with people that has helped millions to exceed their perceived boundaries, worked with others to solve problems and experience success. Project Adventure, an international, non-profit organisation, began in 1971 as an innovative tenth-grade physical education program based in part on the principles of Outward Bound.

Understanding that adventure was more about doing and less about where and what one does, PA's founders developed a program that could be done indoors or on a playing field, accessed by 'students' of all abilities and adaptable to many different time frames.

The program consisted of non-traditional games, warm-ups, trust exercises, group problem-solving activities – many similar to those found in this book – and the use of low and high Challenge Course elements. Students learned to work cooperatively, challenge themselves in a supportive environment, improve self-esteem and learn creative approaches to problem-solving. Yet, all of this occurred without the need to trek in the wilderness, or other such 'high adventure.'

Our goal is simple – 'to bring the adventure home.' Today, with more than 37 years of experience and offices throughout the United States, Australia, New Zealand, Japan and Singapore, Project Adventure has introduced and helped to adapt adventure into literally thousands of academic, corporate, therapeutic and community-based programs.

We maintain a strong belief that a learning environment that utilises adventure and cooperative techniques in a supportive way is an optimal educative experience. Hence, this approach is important for all 'students,' no matter where the 'classroom' is found. Fun is also a major element because, in our experience, people learn more effectively if they enjoy what they are doing. Fun helps to engage people, thereby providing opportunities for growth.

Sharing this way of doing with others is what we do. We continue to create new activities and props; author new and leading-edge publications for the field; offer trainings that help to develop the skills needed to implement this innovative program approach safely and effectively; and provide consultation services to help you develop, apply and maintain a quality program.

Australian English Glossary

It's strange how so many people throughout the world can use a common language (English), and yet often find they can't understand each other. Such is the curiosity of slang, or put lexicographically, the "use of very informal words, phrases or meanings not regarded as standard, or words or phrases used by a specific group of people."

The following is a list of words and phrases that are well understood by me (I have used them in this text) and most true-blue Aussies, but are described and illustrated here for the reference and benefit of our international friends.

Beaut
Short for beautiful and something outstanding of its kind, as in "That was a beaut mistake I just made!"

Cack
Riotous laughter that may cause one to lose their breath, as in "Oh what a cack, did you hear Lionel's joke?"

Cotton On
Understand, usually after some difficulty, as in "He cottoned on to what I told him soon after he hit his head."

Don
To put clothing on one's body, as in "It's cold outside, so don a coat before you leave the house."

Doozy
Something extraordinary, bizarre, or unexpected, as in "That last step was a doozy!"

Full Stop
A complete halt, or period indicating the end of a sentence, as in "There is no more. Full Stop."

Grow Whiskers
Getting old and tired, as in "Whoah, we can't eat that – it's growing whiskers."

Horsey
Resembling the sound of a horse when it sneezes, as in "I let my balloon go to let it splutter and horsey into the wind."

In Situ
In its original position, as in "I liked the couch in situ before we moved it."

Knackered
Very tired, exhausted, as in "I was so knackered, I could barely lift my legs."

Mondo
Large number, lots or way too much to quantify, as in "That is a mondo cup of coffee you're drinking."

Monkey-Grip
When two people join hands, where the fingers of each person curl inside the palm of their partner, and the thumbs sit on top, as in "Research indicates that the monkey-grip is one of the firmest holds you can make with another person."

Mulligan
A golf shot or other attempt that is not tallied against the official score, as in "Let's have a couple of mulligans before we get started."

Nab
To grab, seize or arrest, as in "I have to nab him now before he leaves the office."

Nitty-Gritty
The specific details, the heart of the matter, as in "Let's get down to the nitty-gritty of what happened here."

Office Dog's Body
Person who does all the drudge, mundane, boring tasks, as in "Don't worry, the office dog's body will pick that up later."

Patter
Plausible, persuasive chatter, as in "A good salesperson has their patter down to a fine art."

Penny Drops
As if feeding a coin machine to turn it on, to finally understand something, as in "It was only when I saw the photograph that the penny dropped."

Piff
To propel something through the air, as in "Quick, piff it here and I'll tag him for you."

Pinched
To take something, possibly steal, as in "Who pinched my chips when I wasn't looking?"

Shell-like
Colloquial term for your ear, because it resembles the mother-of-pearl shell, as in "Let me whisper this into your shell-like."

Sod
An informal British term for a youth or man, as in "The poor sod couldn't even buy a drink."

Tid-bits
A choice morsel, especially in terms of gossip or food, as in "I can't eat anymore, do you want the tid-bits?"

Structure of the Book

Working with large groups is a bit like building a house. If you don't start with a good foundation, the house will eventually fall. Or, to twist a universal truth just slightly, if you build it well, they will come.

Thus, I have purposefully structured this book to guide your programming success. The most important bits are at the front, building to ever-higher levels of excitement with each chapter until you reach your much-anticipated peak. And then, it's time to clean up and look to your next 'project.'

THE GROUNDWORK

Your Approach Is Everything

A discussion and check list of the essential ingredients I believe you must have to deliver extraordinary programs – from Go to Whoa – no matter how many people you are working with. It's all in your approach. Full stop.

What's So Special About Large Groups Anyway?

Perhaps you've wondered, but this section identifies why working with large groups is so special and unique when compared to working with small groups.

Essential Tips for Working with Large Groups

Some of the most compelling nuggets of programming wisdom I can offer anyone working with large groups. These tips reflect the subtleties of truly expert facilitation to optimize the good and limit the not-so-good aspects of working with large groups.

Processing Large Group Experiences

A few simple techniques to help you conduct an effective debrief or processing session with a large group, and squeeze even more from your program.

How to Adapt Small Group Activities

How do you transform the fun and enjoyment of a small group activity into an activity suitable for a large group? It's not always possible, but this short section will give you a few pointers.

THE NITTY-GRITTY

Group-Splitting Exercises

Tons of inventive, simple and fun ways to split large groups into smaller groups, beyond the tired and incommodious routine of "Okay, pick a partner."

Ice-Breakers & Energisers

Activities to set the tone, invite people to play, interact and, most importantly, laugh. In my opinion, breaking the 'ice' is the most critical (and often, least prepared) part of a program.

Name-Games

Ideas to tempt your group to learn some names. Tough with large numbers, I know, but the higher the level of name-knowingness, the more fun (and trust) your group will develop.

Interactive Fun Activities

Stacks of fun, interactive and engaging activities that will involve your whole group at the same time. Beyond the pure, unadulterated pleasure of mixing and playing with a large group of people, you are sure to discover lots of intrinsic value in these activities too!

Audience Fun Activities

A selection of my most successful, proven and funnest activities that passionately involve a small group of participants, whom the rest of your group will adore as the 'audience.'

Major Events

These activities will easily run for an hour or two. Think a little preparation, a nice open space, and a few easy-to-get-a-hold-of resources. Then add a lot of people, and you're ready to go. Be prepared, your group may love you for these ideas.

Activity Supplements

Rather than squeezing every detail of certain activities into the main body of the text, I have recorded the solutions, lists and activity templates that accompany these activities here.

CLEANING UP

That part of the book where you wash your hands, and take a moment to consider your next move. This section includes some really useful references that are designed specifically to help you continuously improve your programs.

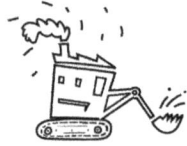

THE GROUNDWORK

In a nutshell

Everything you do and don't do during the 'life' of your program will impact your group. Your program does not start once you have everyone's attention, or resume when your group returns from lunch, or get put on hold when you say "…See you in two hours." Who you are being, and the approach you adopt to deliver the 'whole package' will determine your program's success – both on and off the field.

YOUR APPROACH IS EVERYTHING

When a group of people get together to 'play,' no matter how well-intentioned they may be at the start, they're probably going to play together the way they have always played – with competition and individual heroics very much in the spotlight.

Now, before you get all defensive – there's nothing wrong here! It's not a good or bad situation. But, there is enormous value to consider for a moment why this social phenomenon occurs.

I would argue that this 'way of playing' is not necessarily how people naturally approach play, it's just the way that most of us in the Western culture have been taught to play. Or in other words, it has been learned.

Most games played in today's culture ignore the development of self-confidence, and far from releasing physical aggression, it often promotes it. To illustrate this point, consider for a moment the impact a 'winning is everything' culture has on our language. Some years ago, I was working with a group of university outdoor recreation students – young people who one day aim to be running programs of their own. I asked the students to brainstorm all of the positive and supportive comments they could think of that are a regular part of their vocabulary in their day-to-day 'game' of life, and listed them on the board. From memory, we listed about 20 statements. Then we started listing all of the negative and insulting comments, and in less than three minutes, we added more than 100 different 'put-downs.'

And this does not even begin to consider the game we play inside our heads, our own inner self-talk. We agreed that, on balance, this barrage of statements had to have an impact on our self-image. Even worse, was the realisation that some people may begin to believe what they hear and incorporate these concepts into who they are being, i.e., "I'm a loser."

Whoah – all this is just ten minutes! This simple exercise clearly demonstrated the impact language has on our environment (think, group!). And to think; language is just one element of the chemistry that makes up this peculiar commodity we call 'approach.'

Is Competition Bad?

There's nothing wrong with competition, you know, having winners and losers as such. I believe that competition in and of itself is not bad. I have played competitive tennis on a weekend for most of my life, and I love it.

What is bad is what people allow competition to do to themselves and to others. Or, rephrased in this context – what is bad is the potential harm a group facilitator or leader may allow a competitive approach to do to their group.

As George Leonard says,

"There is nothing wrong with competition in the proper proportion. Like a little salt, it adds zest to the game and to life itself. But when the seasoning is mistaken for the substance, only sickness can follow."

'Winning Isn't Everything
– It's Nothing,'
Intellectual Digest, pp 45-47

Games are like a language – they have incredible potential for connecting people with one another when play is the essence. Unfortunately, when a program is lead and / or approached in an overtly competitive manner, players are prevented from developing a true sense of connectedness with each other, and confidence and community is often destroyed.

And by "competitive manner," I don't just mean the rules of the game and the fact that 'winners and losers' result. I mean everything about your manner – how you have prepared your group and framed their experience, the words you use and your language, imagination and humour, the explicit and implicit goals of the program, and the setting – all of these factors influence the result. Your approach is everything.

Teaching People How to Play

As programs leaders, we have an opportunity to change the rules by which we play – the way in which we invite our groups to play a particular game, as much as our overall program, and indeed, life itself.

If you want your group to come together and be co-operative, inclusive and supportive, then (in most cases) you're going to have to teach them how to play this way. I don't believe it comes naturally. Your group has been, for the most part, conditioned to play in a particular way.

Many people don't even consider playing anymore because they equate play with being left out, not being good enough or feeling like a loser. Your approach will mean the difference between a program appearing as an invitation to share (trust and learn), and one in which many people will feel pressured to participate. Your choice will influence your group's choice.

Are you starting to get that your approach has a huge influence on the success or otherwise of your program? OK, but before you race ahead and start to pick through the variety of awesome activity ideas in this volume, I'd like to offer a checklist of five key ingredients that I believe your approach must reflect to successfully invite people to play. This list will show you how to generate lasting results that will achieve your group's most ambitious needs and revolutionise the way you deliver programs – forever!

Key Ingredients That Invite People To Play

Does your approach to programming:

- Reflect a good sense of humour and spontaneity, where people are allowed and indeed, encouraged to laugh with (as opposed to 'laugh at') one another, suggesting that fun for its own sake is okay?
- Give people the freedom to choose and determine their own levels of participation?
- Use the right activity at the right time, gradually preparing your group for success by presenting a sequence of framed experiences?
- Permit a shared and conscious understanding of how the group is expected to behave, as much as play safely and effectively together?
- Provide opportunities for the group to draw out more from an experience than just having fun?

Put simply, does your approach reflect and uphold choice, fun and discovery all within a valued and carefully sequenced environment? If so, then you are well on the way to 'teaching' your group how to play, and meet their goals.

Project Adventure Philosophies

A series of 'fun' activities played one after the other, however, does not instinctively create a fun and successful experience for everyone. As I've explained, the key to success is the approach you take in the design, framing and delivery of your program – no matter what activities you are presenting – from team building workshops to a basketball clinic, bush-walking to teaching classroom science. The whole package – not just the right activities, but the right approach, and the right preparation – will directly impact how much fun your program creates for everyone, including you.

On the surface, fun seems so simple, but I assure you, it's not always easy. If you find yourself nodding in agreement, let me briefly introduce Project Adventure's simple, yet powerful approach to programming that epitomises the five key ingredients I described above.

Sequencing
Using the right activity at the right time.

Challenge by Choice
Giving people the freedom to choose and determine their own level of participation.

FUNN
A whimsical acronym for Functional Understanding Not Necessary, suggesting that fun for its own sake is okay.

The Full Value Contract
A powerful cultural framework that can help groups to guide their work, manage their behaviours and play together more safely and effectively.

Experiential Learning Cycle
A tool that can help participants draw more from an experience than just having fun, i.e., when you want to crank up the intrinsic side of fun.

Take a look at the Cleaning Up section (page 244) for an expanded discussion of these philosophies.

Putting It Into Practice

Let's consider a few examples of how 'approach is everything.' To reiterate, if you and your program are all about producing supportive, inclusive and positive outcomes, then consider how each of these (real-happened-to-me) teachable moments reflects your understanding of successful programming.

Elimination Games

Presented too early in a program, or too often, games that eliminate people can isolate some (slow, weak, forgetful, etc) people who may have performed poorly in the past with similar activities. Develop a stronger, more supportive atmosphere first so that a higher level of trust may exist within the group to invite more people to play and feel more comfortable to 'look the fool.' Then the 'elimination' is just a part of the game, and not a reflection of life!

You're Out!

How often do we describe the consequences of a penalty with something like "...and if you are too slow or make a mistake, then you have to come into the centre of the circle...""? It is far more powerful and empowering to say "...and if you happen to blurt out the wrong name, or are slower than the person in the middle, it's your turn to have some fun in the centre...."" It's not pedantics, it's all about approach. It's not enough just to say "you are free to choose" at the beginning of the program and then force people to do stuff. You have to walk your talk.

Team Building & Night-Time Activities

I delivered a full-on, intensive team development program for a corporation that enjoyed a really successful day, and then, after dinner, all of the participants returned to their hotel rooms and watched in-house movies – alone! It was like, three steps forward, one step back. Imagine what would be possible if my housing approach matched my program approach. Today, I always recommend shared accommodation, and offer fun, community-building activities in the evening which continue to provide opportunities for my group to connect.

Telling People What to Do versus Issuing An Invitation

One of the most common approaches I see traditional school teachers take when they see a student struggling with a problem is to 'save' them. More often than not, they 'save' the student from who-knows-what, and end up telling or showing them what they have to do to solve the problem. But it's not just teachers, we all do it, some more often than others.

By all means, if someone asks for help (to ask for help can be a huge challenge on its own for some people), or is in danger of hurting themselves, then 'save' them. But in most cases, this is not the situation. A more powerful, empowering approach would be to allow the participant / group to discover the answer for themselves.

Guide them, ask questions which lead to breakthroughs, encourage them, and so on. Consider the difference between asking a group "Do you have any questions.?" and "What questions do you have?" If one can assume that people will have questions to ask, they are more likely to ask them!

This approach subscribes very much to a 'learner-driven learning' methodology as distinguished from 'teacher-driven learning.'

Pick A Partner

Sadly, the instruction to "pick a partner" is too-oft interpreted as "find someone you are attracted to." This thought is as embarrassing as it is open to the anxiety-laden prospect of people feeling left out. There are just too many other fun and non-threatening ways to ask people to get into smaller groups, including pairs, to risk these outcomes. Again, this is a great example of how your approach makes all the difference.

Now, I'm not suggesting that you should never use the words "pick a partner" again. Certainly, as a program develops and your group becomes more comfortable with one another, the panic-inducing reaction to simply 'picking a partner' will diminish. But, with most groups, especially if they have just met each other, you are well advised to avoid the typical "pick a partner" suggestion.

Check out the Group-Splitting Exercises on page 32 for some amusing, often random methods to foster positive-partner-choosing and splitting your large group into small groups.

So, do you think your approach makes a difference? You betcha! Sure there are many awesome activities in this book, ready to open a can of whoopee with your group. But the real gem is in what you have just absorbed.

If you are up for running really healthy and successful programs – no matter how large your group is – I strongly recommend that you embrace the five key ingredients I described above that will unequivocally invite your group to play (trust and learn!).

WHAT'S SO SPECIAL ABOUT LARGE GROUPS ANYWAY?

Here's my take on why working with large groups is so distinctively special.

Energy

The larger the group, the more energy they generate – which means, you don't have to do or say too much to move or motivate the group. You've heard the saying, there's a clown in every group. Well, the larger the group, the more likely you'll have the entire circus turn up. Strangely, large groups tend to find me funnier than smaller groups. The thing is though – I contribute a lot less with large groups, often because I can't get a word in edge-ways! So, I guess it must be the group's own energy that tickles their collective funny bone.

Also, large groups of people invariably do not arrive together, nor all on time. So, another beauty of big groups is that on most occasions, enough people have arrived by starting time to start. Get 'em busy I say, I hate waiting around too.

However, if things don't go the way you plan, the numbers are not in your favour. That's a downside, so at this point, large numbers tend to only exacerbate the anxious feelings you worked so hard in the beginning to hide. Also, if you don't have a good strong voice, or don't have access to a good PA system, you'll lose your voice before recess. Not to mention lose your group, because they can't hear you.

Resources

Large groups consume a lot of stuff – space, time, leaders and equipment! Large groups are fantastic when you plan to lead a series of 'no prop' style activities within an acoustically-perfect indoor stadium. But, for every other occasion, you're up for lots of 'more.'

More props to equip everyone with whatever they need to play with (think issues of not having enough to go around, or worse, not getting it all back at the end). More leaders to spread the load of delivery (think opportunities for fun teamwork, but more effort to involve and communicate effectively). More time because it just takes longer for a larger group to stop playing, or quiet down, or assemble, or move to another spot, etc. More space because, well, ...you get the idea. My advice – factor all of these 'mores' into your large group program.

Safety

It's easy to hide in a large group, because it's true, unlike a small group, one person doesn't stand out as much and there are just too many people to pay particular attention to. Consider the positive impact this fact may have on your program, especially within the context of a fun, interactive and non-threatening program of activities – participants can more comfortably make appropriate choices regarding their level of participation.

For example, in large groups, people who tend to be less outgoing enjoy the fact that there is no particular focus on them as they undertake an activity, because everyone else is busy too. Standing at the back of the group is also a safe place to be, to avoid the potential of being seen or chosen as a 'volunteer.' Simply put, there's safety in numbers.

Of course, the downside is that owing to the sheer size of the group, you may not notice that so-and-so is missing, or is uncomfortable. It is also true that it's harder for you to maintain a watchful eye on everything – there's just too much going on with large groups

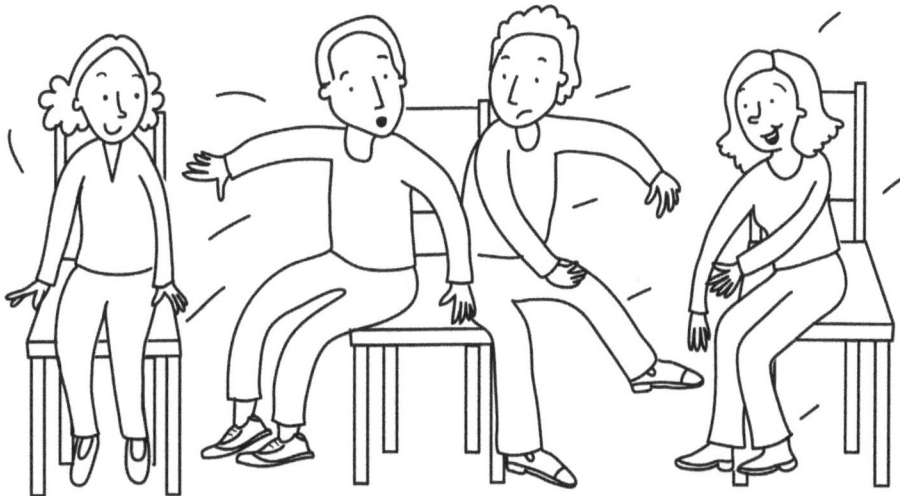

– physically, mentally and emotionally. Being big opens up all sorts of opportunities for distracting behaviour too, including my pet-hate – side-conversations – all under the guise of the 'no-one-will-notice-me' banner.

Anyway, that's what I reckon makes large groups so special. It's now time to explore how you can optimise the good – and limit the not-so-good aspects – of working with large groups.

ESSENTIAL TIPS FOR WORKING WITH LARGE GROUPS

The following tips capture what I believe to be the most useful, practical advice for working effectively with groups no matter what size, but especially if they are large. Note, I said effectively. Anyone can run a program with a big group, but the advice I share below (in no particular order) will move everyone's experience from a so-so time, to a truly rewarding event.

Just Start Playing

One of the surest ways of killing your program right off the bat, is to announce, "Hi, my name is Mark, and I'd like to play a game with you…" To be brutally honest, the best way to ruin a game is to tell your group that you're going to play a game. Just start. Don't fluff about, get them busy as soon as you can. I often leave my intros and name-knowing stuff until much later into the program. And if I'm still waiting for some folks to arrive, I frequently make use of the 'unofficial' start to kick off proceedings – which is simply a ruse to keep people busy.

This advice is just as germane for small groups, but the speed at which a negative thought spreads with a large group is 10 times faster. Don't give it a chance to germinate, and people will be swept along with a more powerful form of contagion – your enthusiasm!

To give you an idea of how it's done, here's an actual excerpt from a recent audio recording:

"Heelllloooooooooo, and welcome. Come on in (waving my hands towards me), don't worry about forming a circle, just bunch on in. <pause> Hi folks, my name is Mark Collard, and welcome to [name of program]. Now (smiling broadly), if you're like me, and you sometimes find yourself standing with a group of people you don't know, you often feel a little self-conscious, right? You look around, and notice that most people seem to have nothing in common with you, or worse, no one appears to be feeling quite as awkward as you. Sometimes, you'll be standing there with your arms crossed, thinking, I'm not going to be forced to do anything. <sniggers as several people uncross their arms> To make those folks who just uncrossed their arms a little more comfortable <more laughter> I invite you all to cross your arms in front of you now. Now, perhaps you've never thought about this before, but you have all just unconsciously divided yourselves into two groups. You either have your left arm crossed over your right, like me. Or, and I have now changed, you have your right arm crossed over your left. If you are a left-armie like me, I would like you to stand over here <pointing to my left> …. and if you are a right-armie, I'd like you to stand over here……"

And in the space of 60 seconds, I have not only started my program, but I have also managed to introduce myself, arouse some laughter, generate some feelings of empathy and not announce a single game!!

Use Pairs

Paired activities – those which require two people to play – are my favorite choice when it comes to working with large groups. First of all, it's hard to be left out of a pair, so it creates lots of 'safety' within a group. Many partnerships doing the same thing also generates lots of energy, which goes a long way to creating success in your program. Also, it is rare for the individual members of large groups to know everybody, so presenting a series of paired-activities in which you frequently invite people to swap partners (see Group-Splitting Exercises later) creates lots of mixing and getting-to-know-one-another moments. And finally, if you discover an uneven number of people in your group – guess what? – it's your turn to play!

Being Heard

Being heard is not just a matter of raising your voice. In fact, I strongly recommend that you don't raise your voice if your group can hear you otherwise.

Imagine for a moment that your voice has a volume dial, ranging from 0 (silent) to 10 (maximum loudness). Now consider that your average volume when speaking with someone in general conversation is a 3 or 4. Here's the thing – commit to addressing your group at levels approximating 5 or 6 on most occasions, and if you ever have to

raise or project your voice, do so at a comfortable 7 or 8 and no more. Save the 9 and 10 for the real emergencies – that's what the voice at 9 or 10 was exclusively designed for. Constantly addressing a large group at 9 or 10 will do two things – one, you will quickly lose your voice, and two, your group will get used to you screaming at them and may gradually talk even louder to be heard over you! It can be a never-ending cycle.

I have found that the most effective volume for addressing my group is approx 5 or no more than 6. Once people get the idea that I am speaking, they quieten down, lean or shuffle in toward me, and then surprisingly, even the largest groups with up to 200 sets of ears can hear me.

Get Their Attention

In my opinion, if you can't be heard or generally have to fight to get the attention of your party, you will find it difficult to work with groups no matter what their size. If this is the case, try some of my favourite attention getters (I 'tips me hat' to many years spent at summer camp, countless programs and tons of public-speaking gigs for providing me with these gems). Some are more appropriate for young people than adults, but all are equally effective.

- Raise your hand, and instruct each group member to raise his or her hand when they see any hands raised. Like my old summer camp leader used to say, "When the hand goes up, the mouth goes shut."

- Say in your normal conversation voice, "If you can hear me, clap once" to invite all those within earshot to follow suit (clap). Then continue with, "If you can hear me, clap three times" (clap, clap, clap). And so on, until the room gets the message. Change the number of claps to gauge the level of listeningness.

- Clap in a pattern – similar to above technique, but this time, you just start clapping a particular beat or tune, and repeat it several times.

- Snap your fingers. Works a treat, but I find my fingers get tired quickly.

- Count down with a loud, "FIIIIVE, FOOOUR, THREEEE...." If you have them trained, by the time you get to three, most of the group will be with you.

- Throw a ball in the air and catch it. Train your group in advance that when the ball is in the air, they can make as much noise as they like, and when the ball is caught, everyone must suddenly fall silent. You will need to repeat this several times to get the attention you desire. Have fun in the beginning when training with several fake throws and drops of the ball.

- Stand up and talk very softly. Very soon, a wave of recognition will flow through the group that says, "Sshhhhh..." Be sure that the initial things you say are nonsense, otherwise, it is highly unlikely that everyone in your group heard your message.

- Simply wait. When the time I'm wasting is not mine, I'll happily stand silently and wait for my group to notice me. It can take a while but is the least costly in terms of energy.

What's the weirdest stunt I've pulled to get my group's attention? Once, with a large corporate crowd, I struggled to get anyone to hear me – so I calmly lied prostrate on the floor. Took only 10 seconds. Hilarious.

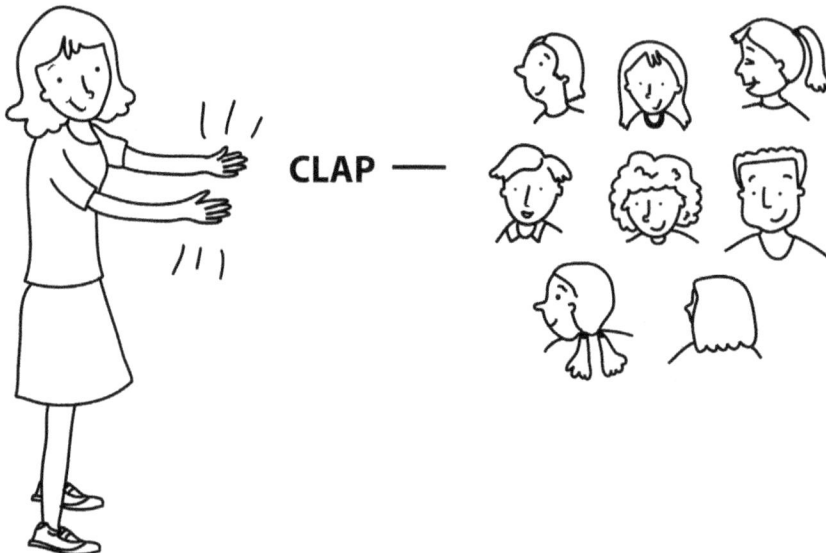

CLAP —

Position Yourself Strategically

Much of the success achieved by an 'expert' (regardless of their field) can be explained by subtlety. In the realm of programming, here are five key subtleties to take serious note of when it comes to strategically positioning yourself in relation to your group.

- Circles are good. Generally speaking, standing as part of a circle, your group has the best chance of not only seeing you, but everyone else in the group. This will lead to engagement and interest. However, hearing you may be another issue. In my experience, once a group numbers 70 or more, this technique starts to grow whiskers.

- Always look into the sun or towards a bright / back-lit background. Yes, it will be more difficult (for you) than if you had the awkward brightness behind you, but if this was the case, you'd end up with a whole lot more people looking anywhere other than at you.

- Stand looking toward the most interesting part of the room / playing field, etc. Again, this strategy attempts to drive the focus toward you as much as possible, and not have to compete with, for example, gorgeous balcony views, television shows, passer-bys, traffic, a meal being prepared, etc.

- Tell a secret. I love lowering my voice and inviting my group to "bunch on in" around me. The closer my group gets, the more energy and intimacy they will generate, the less I have to project my voice, and most importantly, the more excitement I can build into my patter.

- On a windy day, stand so that the wind may carry your voice toward your group.

Factor In More of Everything

As discussed on page 18, large groups consume more of everything. Plan accordingly. The activities will take more time than you expect – allow at least an extra 20% than you would for 'smaller' groups. You will need more equipment to share around, especially if there is a risk of breakage or spillage – have more on hand than you think is necessary. You will need more people or leaders to help you be heard, control the crowd, distribute and gather things, etc.

Break It Up

Owing to issues of attention-deficit, distractions, and the possibility that maybe not everyone can hear you, break everything you need to say into little chunks. Tell them only what they need to know when they need to know it. And apply the well-known saying – a picture tells a thousand words. Provide lots of practical examples of what to do and what it looks like. This tip alone saved me countless hours of translation with many non-English speaking populations. Invite a volunteer from the crowd – this is a sure-fire way to engage your group.

Your goal should be to brief an activity and not have to field any questions at the end. However, don't be afraid to start an activity if you feel that a few people are confused. Oftentimes, these people will get it once they see others doing it. And if not, you can respond accordingly while everyone else is occupied.

Preserve the Adventure

To follow on from this last point, maintain as much mystery and adventure (i.e., unanticipated outcomes) in your program / approach as possible. Half of the fun of a truly successful program is found in the rudiments of surprise and discovery of what you do, and don't do. Everything from inviting a volunteer from the crowd before you have described what they are being asked to do, through to keeping the punch line (so to speak) of your activity right to the end. This approach will engage people, and build excitement. And, when facilitated well, engagement promotes discovery and learning. It can often be the difference between "What are we doing next?" and "Oh no, not that again."

This tip applies equally across the board, regardless of how big your group is, but especially with large groups because you are dealing with a much more forceful energy. Large groups possess a life of their own, where you can be riding the crest of a wave one minute, and smashing into the surf the next. Remember, play in its purest, most innocent form is not often experienced by many people these days. So any hint of 'we're-about-to-play-something' may cause some people to run in the other direction.

Aim to pique their interest, invite them forward, tease them almost. And before they know it, your group is more likely to be doing something that, if they had known what it was in advance, they would not have come to so easily. And, this is just a guess, but I reckon that most of these initially reluctant people are grateful in the end.

Hydrate, Hydrate, Hydrate

Your voice is a finely-tuned instrument, and one of your most vital tools as a program leader. If you don't look after it, it will not be there when you need it. Short of advising you to check into a voice-care workshop, I strongly recommend that you sip and drink lots of water – during ALL of your program. You should be drinking at least two litres (half gallon) of water every day anyway, so plan to drink a whole lot more if you are exercising your voice. I also recommend that you drink copious amounts of water before the program starts, because it can take at least 30 minutes for the water to hit your vocal folds. If your voice hurts after a program, this can only point to one of three issues – not drinking enough water, over-taxing your voice (read 'Being Heard' tips above), or not breathing properly (in which case, you'll need to seek professional advice).

Use Innovative Group-Splitting Exercises

When I was at school, I hated the typical "1, 2, 3, 4, 1, 2, 3, 4, 1, 2, …" count off, not to mention the dreaded 'pick two captains' scenario (yes, I was always picked last!). These self-esteem crushing exercises are not fun, and are not particularly good at creating random, fairly even groupings either. Commit to using a variety of innovative and fun methods to separate your large group into smaller groups. They generate energy, and often lots of laughter in the process. In some cases, the group does not even recognise that they are being split up until it's too late – perfect for interrupting those hard-to-crack cliques.

Sneak a peek at pages 32 to 41 for lots of fun, creative and totally engaging group-splitting ideas.

Be Adaptable

Finally, let go of the idea that everything will run perfectly. It won't. The 'program' will always require your constant attention to changes that occur within the group (and not necessarily for the worse). And that's OK, provided you don't stress over it – simply adjust your program on the run, keeping your group's goals in mind at all times. This advice is worthy of all program providers, but especially for those who work with large groups, because based on my experience, the mantra 'stuff happens' multiplies in proportion to the number of people.

PROCESSING LARGE GROUP EXPERIENCES

For some, leading an effective debrief is about as scary as leading a really large group of people. So, it's not surprising that when you combine these two activities, many people choose to run the other way.

A debrief, or processing session, regardless of the number of people involved, need not be panic-inducing. To learn about a really simple debrief model, take a look at my discussion of the Experiential Learning Cycle at the back of this book, page 251. This model will help you to sequence your 'process' conversation and help you squeeze even more out of your program.

Then, armed with a really effective processing model, take your pick from the list of really simple techniques I discuss below to help you process the,

otherwise daunting task, of processing a large group's experience.

One of the greatest killers to an effective processing session (with any size group, but especially large groups) is a distinct lack of energy. Which is often the same as saying, no one is feeling 'safe.' Frequently, this occurs because the facilitator has asked for too much, too soon with too many people at once. Nurture the energy of your group first, get people comfortable talking in a safe environment, and then build on that success.

The first bunch of ideas I share below subscribe to this philosophy, while the remainder are just good large group management techniques.

Paired-Shares

Simply ask your group to turn to one or more people around them, and discuss a particular topic, question or statement that you pose. You will immediately generate lots of energy. Even if only half of the group actually focuses on what they have been asked to discuss, it won't matter because all of the conversations will lift the group's energy for sharing. See page 43 for more ideas.

Whip Around

Useful for numbers of up to forty or so people, this technique invites individuals to quickly share a word or phrase only in response to a question posed to the group. Having formed a circle, you pose a question or statement to your group, and then 'whip around' the circle in whatever direction, inviting each person's response. This technique is quick, easy to administer and ideal for groups who suffer from dominant or loud participants.

If you determine that the information garnered from these words or phrases is too brief, whip around a second time, asking each person to 'use' their word in a sentence to explain why they chose that word the first time around.

Back to Back

Ideal in pairs, but you could involve three or four people. Ask your group to form into pairs, standing back to back with their partners. Then, within earshot of everyone, pose a question, and instruct participants to face their partners and respond to them as soon as you say, "GO." Allow 30 to 60 seconds for an adequate response, and then yell "BACK TO BACK." The partners either resume their original back-to-back stance with their partner, or, you may invite everyone to find a new partner. Repeat several times, each question becoming increasingly deep.

Small Groups

Divide your group into smaller groups of roughly five to eight people (beyond eight, and some folks struggle to be heard). Invite each group to circle up, and then pose a series of questions for each group to discuss. If you wish, ask the group to nominate a 'scribe' to record the group's responses, for possible sharing with the large group. Or, provide a list of questions on a sheet of paper so that each group can write their answers.

Another alternative that builds energy is to supply just one question on a sheet of paper. For example, one person from each group collects the first sheet from you, returns to their group to discuss and record the group's responses, and then someone new comes back to you to receive the second question, and so on.

Thumbs Up Ranking

Ask each person in your group to simply extend one or more fingers on their hand to indicate their rank or assessment of a certain criteria you pose. For example, "On a scale of 1 to 5, five being highest, rate how well you think the group communicated in this exercise." This works best in a circle, where everyone's opinion can be seen. It's simple, non-verbal, and will give you a quick guide as to where the group is at.

If you feel that some folks may be influenced by the opinion (ranking) of others, first ask that everyone closes their eyes and then extend their fingers. This technique won't necessarily eliminate last minute changes once eyes have re-opened, but it will keep most people honest.

The Plenary

Having generated lots of energy by sparking dozens of little conversations or input from your group, form a large circle or bunch them all in together, and invite some general (plenary) sharing. Questions such as "Can someone share one thing that was discussed with his or her partner that seemed particularly significant?" or "Based on what we have all heard, could someone suggest what we may have learned from this experience?"

The fact that you have 'warmed up' your group will make this technique work far more effectively than if you launched into it too early.

Observers

This technique is as much a useful large group program design option as it is a wonderful processing tool. Divide your group in two. Depending on your numbers, and the nature of the activity, you may choose an equal 50/50 split, or simply nominate a small group of folks to separate from the larger group. The idea is for one group to perform the activity, while the other observes what happens with a view to providing some guided feedback at the conclusion.

For young people, I suggest you prepare a list of attributes for the observers to monitor. You may also need to provide guidance for offering constructive feedback. If time permits with 50/50 splits, it's often fascinating to explore what happens when you ask each group to swap roles, so the original observers become the active participants.

HOW TO ADAPT SMALL GROUP ACTIVITIES

After playing a fantastic activity with a small group, people often ask, "Will it work with a large group?" Well, they say you can't fit a square peg into a round hole. The same belief is generally held about 'super-sizing' small group activities for large groups. But, I'm not convinced.

Here are a few pointers that will help you explore the possibilities of squeezing as much, if not more, fun from a small group activity with a large group.

Multiple Small Groups

The simplest solution is to divide your large group and establish multiple small group activities. Beware that this strategy may also require extra facilitators, but not always. The activity of several small groups can often be managed successfully by one person (you).

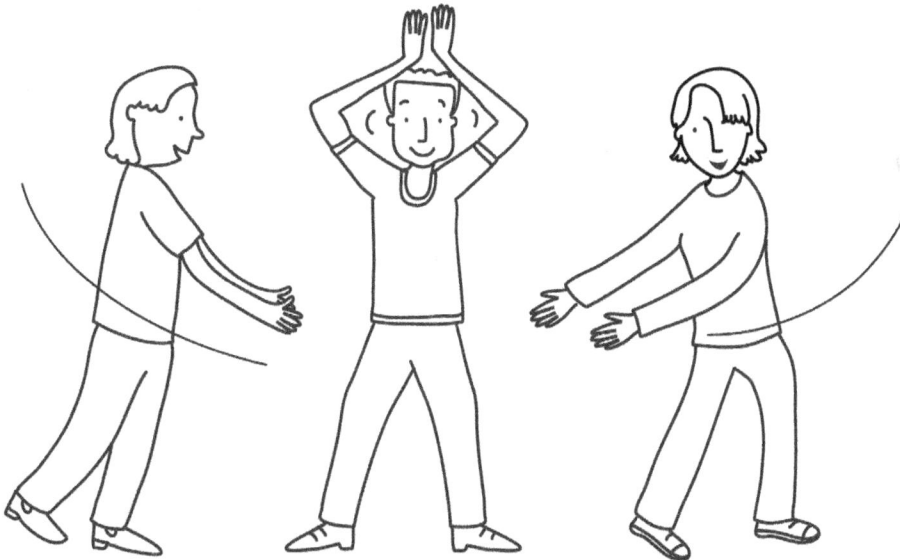

A large majority of the activities in this book are designed to keep your group – your whole group – active and / or engaged at the same time. For a few activities, you may need to divide your large group into smaller groups to achieve this goal. As such, the activity descriptions (which follow) will describe when this is necessary, and how to do it successfully.

Observers

Divide your group so that, say, half of your group actively participates while the other half observes. Now, I don't just mean 'sit out' – that's not much fun. Give this observation group something productive to do. For example, invite them to take note of certain interactions of the playing group, per-haps with a view to providing feedback at the conclusion of the activity. Then – this is the interesting part – switch the groups. Now it's time for the observers to become the players. In my experi-ence, the observers often behave the same way as the group they observed, despite having just offered valuable feedback about said behaviours to the latter!

Keep It Simple

In most cases, activities that involve two, three or four people, or require no equipment at all to play, are ideal for large groups. Space permitting, you can never have too many pairs, triads or quads. Also, plenty of 'no prop' style activities means that you will always have everything that you need.

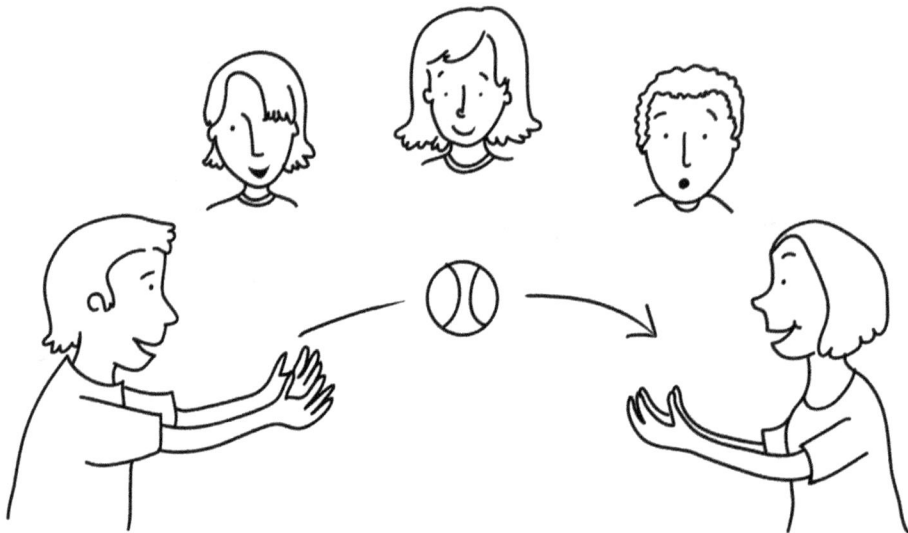

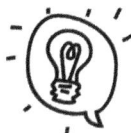

THE NITTY-GRITTY

This section is jam-packed full of the best and most fun activity ideas I have come across that work with large groups of people. In fact, they will work with pretty much any size group.

From the simplest of ice-breakers to a series of high-energy, full-on events that will occupy your people for an hour or two, this range of highly successful sure-fire large group activities is for you and yours to enjoy.

The activities have been broadly categorised according to their best use. However, before you dive head-long into the following pages, it is useful to understand what distinguishes each type of activity from the others.

ACTIVITY GROUPING

Group-Splitting Exercises

Activities that split large groups into smaller groups.

- Creative / random / non-traditional splits
- Simple instructions
- Generally rapid execution

Ice-Breakers & Energisers

Activities that set the tone, and invite people to interact in a non-threatening manner

- Fun and laughter is normally a major component.
- Success-oriented
- Minimal verbal and decision-making skills required
- Stimulate energy and attention.
- 1 to 15 minutes of play

Name-Games

Activities that encourage and enable people to learn one another's names

- Fun and laughter is key.
- Emphasis on effort, rather than results
- Set within a cooperative and supportive environment
- 2 to 15 minutes of play

Interactive Fun Activities

Activities that provide an opportunity for group members to interact, play, trust and learn

- Fun and laughter is normally a major component.
- Emphasis on whole group participation / interaction
- Success-oriented, not win / lose
- 10 to 30 minutes of play

Audience Fun Activities

Activities that provide an opportunity for a small number of people to entertain the rest of their group

- Focus on fun, laughter and amusement
- Active participation is optional.
- Audience participation is encouraged.
- 15 to 60 minutes of play

Major Events

Activities that will occupy and involve a group for long periods

- Fun and interaction is key
- Typically require intense preparation, staff and equipment needs
- 1 to 2 or more hours of play

Now, it often happens that folks believe that because an activity fits into one category, it cannot be used elsewhere in their program sequence. Or worse still, some believe that the way I present the activities here is the way that they should be played. In a word, wrong.

For some activities, this may be the case, but for most, this is not a truth. A simple tweaking of a rule here, or the introduction of a limitation there, and voila! you have a new activity.

For example, consider Categories (page 45). It is so versatile, it can be used as an ice-breaker for at least 15 or 20 minutes to mix people, generate lots of laughter and create a really supportive atmosphere. Yet, using just one 'category' to create four random teams to play a large interactive activity, it becomes a simple Group-Splitting Exercise.

Or, consider the awesome interactive activity of Finger-Snaps (page 155). This activity is typically presented as a series of high energy, dynamic, spirited games, but it can also be exclusively designed as a group problem-solving activity.

The beauty of the activities contained within these pages is that they can be played in so many different ways. This book presents only a common description of the game, followed by at least one or two variations.

Remember, as soon as you have tried the activity – it's yours, and then with a little poetic license, you can change it to meet the needs of your group.

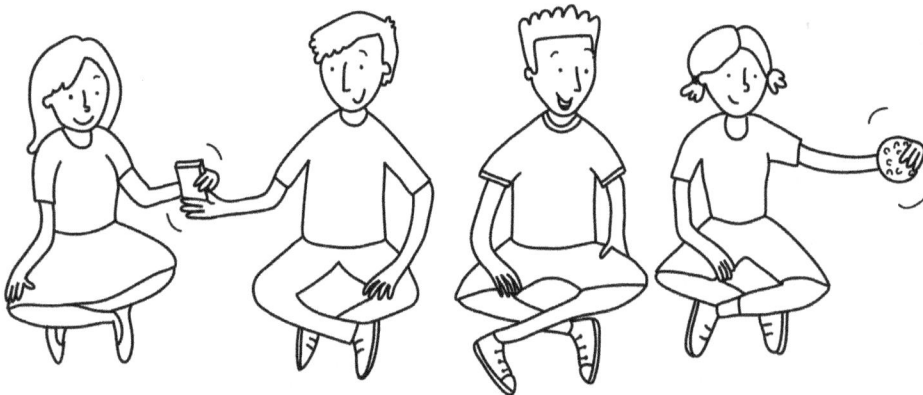

DESCRIPTION FORMAT

Each activity is described, for the most part, using the following characteristics:

AT A GLANCE

Designed to give you a basic idea of what the activity is and looks like in one breath

WHAT YOU NEED

General requirements of space and equipment needed (if any) to run the activity successfully and safely

Optional equipment you will need if you choose to vary the activity

Estimated time you can expect the activity will run for (not including the briefing, or variations)

WHAT TO DO

A play-by-play description of how you could choose to introduce the activity; everything you need to know to get you started. Much of my language will be presented as if I were speaking directly to a group, but I pull out of the group context often to put on my 'leader's hat.'

VARIATIONS

Suggestions from simple rule changes to complex variations of the basic activity. For most activities, the sky's the limit.

As a further guide, the illustrations aim to capture the essence or critical elements of each activity, to make it a little easier for the activities to jump off the page for you.

A Note on Safety

It is important to consider the safety aspects of each activity, and to address the concerns that each one presents. Remember, the activities presented here involve the same risk management concerns as any program: being aware of environment, hazards and terrain, group ability, readiness, clothing and so on.

When briefing the activities in this book, point out hazards in the play area that may cause harm, such as dips in terrain. If grass is wet and slippery, be especially wary of doing running games. Issues of terrain and environment are one of the reasons that games produce more injuries than their more drama-packed adventure-based program cousins!

Additionally, be aware of medical and physical issues in your group that may cause a particular activity to be inappropriate. Shoulder injuries, sprained ankles and back problems are common, and can be exacerbated given the nature of some activities. Challenge by Choice is more than an essential cornerstone in program quality; it's also an important tool for keeping people safe. Make sure that participants understand their choices.

Finally, be on the look-out for group readiness. Do participants have the skills to perform the activity? Has a particular participant been shown to be somewhat unsteady on his or her feet? Lack of readiness can also put a group at risk. Follow the guidelines for sequencing to increase the chances of a safe experience for all.

GROUP-SPLITTING IDEAS

Tucked within this publication are a myriad of activities that will keep your whole group together and active doing the same thing at the same time. As such, once your group has assembled, they are ready to go.

But, there are many large group activities that work more effectively if you, first, split your aggregation into smaller groupings. Indeed, one of the first things we often want to do when faced with an army of people (other than run away) is to separate them into more manageable parcels. This strategy alone can be a very successful way to 'warm up' your group, and in particular, build their skills gradually working from smaller to larger units.

Also, keep in mind that once split, these smaller groups are ripe for sharing, which is often difficult to achieve with large groups. A method I often employ is to split the group several times for the purposes of interaction, and every now and then, ask the current assembly of small groups to respond to one or more questions I pose. See Paired Shares on page 43 for some great examples.

All right, so how do you divide your group?

Let's say you've got 50 people, and need five groups – that'll make ten people per group, right? Yes, but how do you decide which ten go into which group? The composition of each group, and the manner in which the members are chosen can make a big difference to the outcome of an activity – not to mention how each member may feel about their belongingness (take a look at 'Your Approach Is Everything' on page 14). Take, for example, two traditional group-splitting methods that I recall my teacher using in high school (and many years on, I know they still get used):

(a) The teacher / leader picks two (or more) 'captains' and the captains pick their own teams. Just fine if you're friends with one of the newly appointed. But, an unmitigated disaster if you are – like me – one of the smallest, less-coordinated kids on the block. The result – an argument mounted by each team at the end of the choosing as to why the other team should have to take me. Like I said, not a good self-esteem building exercise.

(b) Then there's the old count-off method – 1, 2, 3, 4, 1, 2, 3, 4, and so on. Have you ever noticed how people will often move their place in the line (ahead of the counting) just so that they will get a number they want, i.e., that which matches their friends'? Or worse, short of branding a number on people's foreheads, how do you police who is in whose group anyway?

Sure, these methods can work. But, rarely do they produce balanced teams (in terms of players, skill levels or both), and are about as much fun as they are self-esteem building exercises – not! So – ta da! – here is a collection of some of my favourite group-splitting methods, each of them inspired by a number of fun variations.

Consider the size of your group, the number of smaller groups you want to establish, and how much time you would like to devote to the splitting process. This third factor is helpful because many of the following ideas (all with tons of variations) are fun to play just for their own delectation. All you need is some open space to spread folks out, and as many of them as you can muster.

Clumps
Snappy Partners
Psychic Handshake
Pick a Number Out of a Hat
Puzzle Pieces
Do It Yourself

In addition to the exercises above, I strongly encourage you to check out Categories (page 45) as another sure-fire large-group splitting, ice-breaking activity. Enjoy!

CLUMPS

Zany, fast-paced energiser designed to mix people frequently

AT A GLANCE

People quickly form a series of temporary groups matching the number called by the leader.

WHAT YOU NEED

5 - 10 mins

WHAT TO DO

This is so simple, yet so good. Gather your group around you, and explain that, in a moment, you will shout out a number – any number from, say one to ten (the bigger your group, the bigger you can make the top end). Immediately, everyone must form a group consisting of that number of people. In my experience, groups get very huggy at this point, and form little fortresses with their bodies to prevent others from joining their little huddle.

Naturally, you will often get a few poor souls left over, the so-called remainder, if we speak in the language of long division. At this moment, you have several options. You can eliminate these folks, move them to the side, and continue with the next shouted number, and so on until you get the lucky 'winners.' This is fine; however, I think it's best to simply shout another number. It keeps the energy up, is much less competitive, and more fun for everyone. And the look on the faces of the 'dejected' when they hear the next number called ('I'm saved') is priceless.

Move from five to three, then up to nine and back down to four so that a high degree of mixing occurs. Shout "ONE!" just to see what happens.

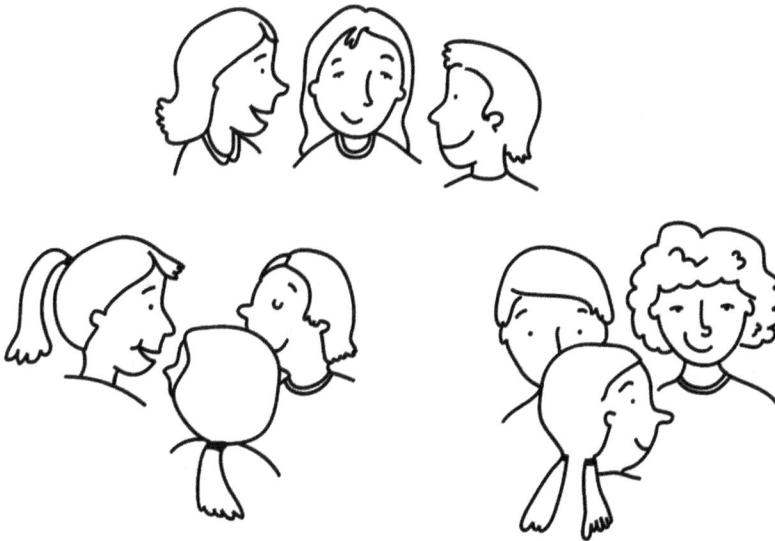

Variations

- Add the proviso that when a new number is called, a person cannot form a group with anyone who was in their previous group (as much as is possible). This tweaking of the rules will spoil the plans of those crafty individuals who prefer to stick together, simply opting to ebb and flow in terms of their membership number at any point in time.

- Form a group according to a simple, easily-accessible category, such as dark-coloured tops, brand of running shoes, gender, colour of eyes, etc. Similar to Categories on page 45.

- Once formed, instruct the newly-created groups to use their collective bodies to make the shape of a letter of the alphabet, or numeral, or object, e.g., table, house, car, etc.

SNAPPY PARTNERS

Some of the quickest and easiest ways to invite people to find a partner, or a group

AT A GLANCE
Individuals find partners according to a random category called by the leader.

WHAT YOU NEED
Deck of playing cards (optional)
10 secs - 2 mins

WHAT TO DO
As described in an earlier section, there is nothing worse than being asked to "find a partner" as you stare into a sea of unknown and quite frightening new faces. It's much easier if you – the facilitator – direct the traffic in the beginning, to diminish a lot of that initial anxiety.

Forming Pairs

There are literally millions of 'categories' you or your group can think of to divide into pairs. No longer do you have an excuse to just say, "Okay, pick a partner." Besides, it's not half as much fun.

Ask your group to find another person who has the same or similar:

- Colour top, pants, socks, underwear, etc
- Type of shoes
- Month of birth, or zodiac sign
- Length or colour of hair
- Height, or size of hands, feet, thumb, ears, etc
- Colour of eyes
- Number of letters, syllables or vowels in their name
- Number of pieces of jewellery being worn
- Favourite car, animal, colour, ice-cream flavour, etc

Here are a few more that require a little more explanation:

- Form a circle facing inward, and on your command, ask everyone to "LOOK DOWN" at the ground, and then on your command, "LOOK UP" directly and purposefully to the eye level of another randomly-chosen group member. If two people happen to look at each other (i.e., by chance), they depart the scene as newly-formed partners, the circle contracts, and the pairing continues.

- With hands behind their backs, everyone extends a certain number of fingers on one (or two) hands. Once ready, ask everyone to reveal their variously extended digits in front of them so that others can see them – the task is to find another person with the same number of exposed fingers.

- Same as above, but ask that only a thumb or pinky finger is extended.

- Ask each person in your group to think of three (or whatever number of groups you need) animals. In one huge cacophonic symphony, ask each person to rapidly and loudly make the sound of all three (or whatever number) animals for roughly ten seconds. Then, ask everyone to shut their eyes, imagine that all but one of the animals have run away, and when they next open their eyes, they are to make only the noise of the animal they have imagined is left remaining (i.e., it is presumed that not everyone will imagine the same animal). Similar creature sounds are the cue for partnership.

- Form one straight line – according to a random fit, or by way of a particular criteria such as height, date of birth, the last two digits of home telephone numbers, etc – and then fold the resulting line in the middle so that each person ends up facing another person to become partners.

- Each person sings out loud the sound of the first vowel of their name, and seeks an equally harmonic partner, or partners as the case requires. Similar to Vowel Orchestra, see page 46.

Splitting Into Two or More Teams

Want just two, three or more teams? Try these out for size. The more 'random' methods described may not always give you a scientifically equal split. But, it will often come close, and more importantly, your group will have had some fun along the way. Balance the teams as you see fit.

Ask your group to:

- Stand next to a friend / someone they know. Instruct one member of the pair to kneel down, and the other to remain standing. Then, ask all those who are standing to move to one side, and voila, you have two even teams. And, as a side-benefit, you have may have separated problematic friends / cliques.

- Same as above, but ask one partner to put their hands on their head, while the other puts their hands on their hips.

- Form a pair (by using one of the earlier methods), and then join up with another pair to form a group of four, and then this combination joins with another quad to produce a group of eight, etc.

- Find other group members who possess the same attributes of:

  - How they cross their arms – left over right, or right over left

  - House or phone numbers – odd and even

- The second letter of their first and last names – both letters are vowels, or one or both are consonants to produce two or three teams
- The playing card they hold – randomly distribute one or more decks of cards (everyone needs just one card to hold). Brilliant for splitting into countless number and size of groupings (pairs, teams, 50 / 50 splits, etc). For example:
  - Colour of card (red and black)
  - Odds / evens
  - Picture / non-picture
  - Suit (Clubs, Diamonds, Hearts & Spades)
  - Two, three or four of a kind
  - A winning Poker combination, e.g., flush, straights, etc.

- Initially form into small teams of whatever number of groups you want to create, e.g., let's say you want four groups, you ask for teams of four people. Then ask each team to create an 'object' where each person assumes the role of one part. Once formed, you ask each person assuming a particular part (from each team) to join the same group. Here are some suggested objects and parts:
  - Animal – head, body, legs, tail, ears, etc
  - Vehicle – wheels, chassis, headlights, seats, engine, etc
  - Band – lead singer, bass guitar, drummer, pianist, etc
  - Burger – meat, cheese, lettuce, tomato, sauce, etc.

PSYCHIC HANDSHAKE

A really FUNN, random method of forming a specific number of groups

AT A GLANCE
People shake hands a fixed number of times to determine the group they belong to.

WHAT YOU NEED
3 - 5 mins

WHAT TO DO
Begin by asking everyone in your group to think of a number, and keep it to themselves. Your choice of number will be determined by the number of small groups you wish to create. So, if you want four groups at the end of this exercise, ask them to think of the numbers 1, 2, 3 or 4.

The idea is for everyone who is thinking of the same number to find one another and gather in one spot. But, unless your group has some sort of extra sensory perceptors at work, I would suggest they will need some further instructions to help them find their designated group. This is where the fun is.

With a number in mind, invite each person to approach another and immerse themselves in a very friendly shaking of hands. Each person will literally shake their own hand (read, arm as well) corresponding to the number they are thinking of, and so will their partner. The key to this banter is for each person to hold their arm firm when he or she accomplishes the required number of shakes. So, if you are thinking 'three' and I'm thinking 'two,' we will happily shake one another's hands for the first two shakes, and then suddenly my arm and hand will go stiff, and prevent any further mutual shakes. At this juncture, it will be obvious from the level of grunts and laughter that emanate from you as you struggle with my 'holding firm' position that we are not on the same wavelength and belong in different groups.

It's a good idea to demonstrate what the 'shaking-of-hands' and 'holding-firm' positions look like – in front of everyone before you say "GO" to give everyone a clue and a chance to giggle at what is really a very FUNN exchange.

Suggest to your group that it is most effective if they remain silent throughout the frenetic shaking period. That is, no talking, but laughter is permitted. Also, a few smart folks will think to indicate with their out-stretched fingers, or by clapping, the number they are thinking of. Applaud their ingenuity, but suggest that it's more fun to stick to the shaking.

Variation

Same set-up, but blind-folded.

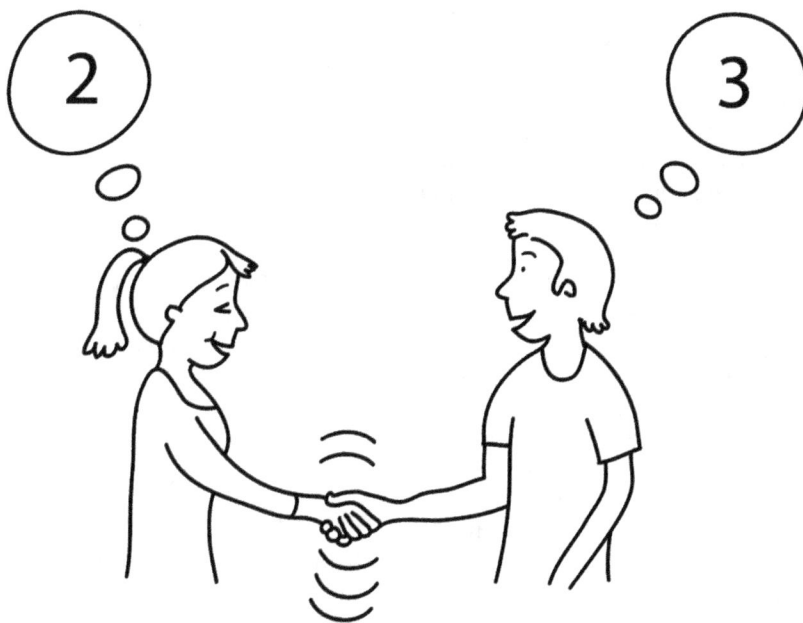

PICK A NUMBER OUT OF A HAT

Some fun, new possibilities for a 'golden-oldie'

AT A GLANCE

People form groups according to the 'category' or 'object' listed on a piece of paper they pull randomly from a hat or other receptacle.

WHAT YOU NEED

Paper, pen and receptacle of sorts
1 - 5 mins

WHAT TO DO

You will need to prepare a little in advance for this group-splitting technique. Find a large receptacle – such as an empty tin can, or a hat – and collect (or cut) as many small pieces of paper as you have people in your group.

Next, you need to decide on a theme that all the pieces of paper will have in common, and then a list of unique identities within that theme. For example, let's say you are looking to form ten groups out of 90 people. You could choose animals as your theme (or any one of the ideas listed below), then list ten different types of animals such as lions, bears, eagles, etc. Write the name of each animal on nine pieces of paper (i.e., each group will have nine players in it). Perhaps fold the pieces of paper up a little (to prevent sneaky hand-picked glances), stuff them all in a big tin can, and you're ready to go.

As you distribute the pieces of paper, ask your group not to show them to other people, nor tell what is written on them. It's a secret! Then, once all of the pieces have been handed out, explain what it is they have to do. Basically, the goal is for everyone to find other looks-or-sounds-like-me people to form a group.

Here are a few ideas that will help to inspire some fun group-sorting banter.

Numbers

Announce your number to the world, or use out-stretched fingers, or even claps to indicate your number.

Shake your hand with another person (as you greet them) according to your number (see Psychic Handshake on page 36).

Animals

Make the sound of the animal (be sure to use animals that have audible sounds or calls).

Mime or act the look of the animal.

Word Associations

Announce your 'word' or simply show your piece of paper, as you mingle about the group, and try to find other people with:

- The same 'word;' or

- A word that is typically associated with your word, e.g., peanut + butter, coca + cola; or

- An object that fits within a particular category, e.g., some folks may be holding 'Cadillac,' 'Holden,' and 'Ford' (make of car), while others in the group hold 'rose,' 'tulip,' or 'daffodil' (type of flower).

Joke & Punch-line

Write a series of jokes or riddles on one set of cards and the corresponding punch-lines on another set. Mix them well and distribute. Use several of the same joke / punch-line, or as many unique jokes as you have people. Once everyone has located their other half, read the jokes outloud.

Action Oriented

Demonstrate the action written on the piece of paper, i.e., everyone who performs the same action is in the same grouping. For example:

- Hop on particular leg
- Jump
- Skip
- Crawl
- Clap your hands
- Whistle a tune
- Scratch my back
- Pull my ear
- Tickle me
- Hold my hand

Hum Dinger

Hum the tune of a popular song or nursery rhyme, etc.

Whistle the tune of a popular song or nursery rhyme, etc.

Sweet Thing

Rather than paper, distribute lollies. Ask people to eat the lolly – such as a jellybean – and divide up according to the colour of their tongue.

OK, so what if you don't know how many people are coming? This is especially true for large conference type gatherings, or public events.

Theory would suggest that if the pieces of paper are sufficiently mixed, each team will have roughly the same number of members, regardless of how many people attend. But, if your activity relies on each team having a specific number of people, I recommend strategically releasing more pieces of paper as more people arrive. For example, let's say you need teams of ten people, and you anticipate that 120 people could arrive at the most. Make up 12 categories of ten things and distribute sufficient pieces to fill, say, six teams in the beginning. Then, as more people arrive, add a new 'team' of ten pieces to the tin. If you do this next step twice, you will end up with eight teams of approx ten people, rather than 12 teams of seven people or so (if you had distributed all of the 12 teams at the start).

PUZZLE PIECES

A really creative way for people to mix with one another, and find their grouping

AT A GLANCE

People use their randomly distributed puzzle piece to complete a jigsaw and locate their group.

WHAT YOU NEED

Set of pre-made jigsaw puzzles (one per group)

1 - 10 mins

WHAT TO DO

You'll need to either purchase a set of pre-fabricated blank cardboard jigsaw puzzle sets, or simply make up a set of puzzles for yourself from coloured sheets of cardboard. In each case, you will want one complete puzzle set for every group you wish to form, and ideally the same number of puzzle pieces as you have members in a group.

Once the puzzles have been selected or created, place all of the pieces into a big bag, mix them up, and when your group has assembled, ask each person to select one piece. Now, instruct each person to find everyone else who holds a piece of the same puzzle, with a view to re-building the puzzle.

Try to make each of the puzzles very unique, and quite distinct in appearance to all the others, i.e., no two pieces should look alike, nor should one piece fit into the frame of another puzzle. One easy way to achieve this is to paint the back of each puzzle with a unique colour, or to use a unique image.

A word of caution – do not make the puzzle too difficult to assemble. Timing will vary, but anything more than five to ten minutes is too long, and will start to diminish the time you had prepared for the 'main event' – the reason for wanting small groups in the first place.

Variation

The puzzle, once it is put back together, could reveal a written clue that provides the group's first activity instructions.

DO IT YOURSELF

The easiest group-splitter of the lot

AT A GLANCE

You allow people to form their own groups.

WHAT YOU NEED

1 - 2 mins

WHAT TO DO

Not much really. Simply ask your group to split according to their own needs and wishes, into as many groups as you command. On most occasions, you will want an even number of players in each 'team' so this will likely be the only boundary the group has to respect.

However, while this option is very attractive insofar as it does not involve much work on your part, I do suggest the exercise will benefit from some further boundaries of your choosing. Otherwise, you could end up with largely un-even teams (in terms of numbers, as well as expertise, experience, gender, etc), the reinforcement of 'cliques' or a group of people off to the side who are not wanted by anybody!

It's a good thing to 'empower' our groups programmatically when possible, but there are times when we need to provide them with a little guidance. To help achieve a more balanced, yet random selection of team members, propose that the group-splitting process respects a set criterion, for example, an even distribution of male / female, age, background, expertise, etc.

When framed correctly, this method will work more often than not. However, if you choose to go this way, be prepared that the group may neglect your good intentions, in which case, you will have no other choice than to proceed with the groupings they create.

ICE-BREAKERS & ENERGISERS

These activities provide an opportunity for the members of your group to begin to feel comfortable with one another. Even if the people know each other pretty well, ice-breakers always start your program off with a few laughs.

Ice-breakers and energisers typically feature:

- Fun as a major component
- Lots of non-threatening interaction
- Success-oriented activity
- Minimal verbal and decision-making skills
- 1 to 15 minutes of play

I have categorised this section into three further activity distinctions, regarding the number of people involved and the general thrust of the exercise. Within each distinction, there is a sequence reflecting a gradual increase in the level of interaction, challenge and / or exertion required.

**Ice-Breakers, Mixers &
Getting-To-Know-You Activities**

Paired Shares
Categories
Vowel Orchestra
Jelly Bean Trade
Spectrums
Mapping
Signature Bingo
Nonsense Numbers
Vortex
Mintie Game
Who Am I?
Acronyms
Wordles
Alphabet Equations
Comfort Circle
Sit Down If...
All My Neighbours
Do You Love Your Neighbours?
Five Clues
Categories with a Twist
Snowflake
Talking Behind Your Back
Ace of Spades

Partner Activities

Thumb Wrestling In Stereo
ESP
Spot the Difference

Bouncey Bouncey
Off Balance
Finger Fencing
Toe Tag
Squat Thrust
Moon Walking
Human Spring

Large Group Energisers

Clapping Game
Gotcha
Galloping Hands
Beat the Bunny
Fill the Space
Stop & Go
Mr & Mrs Wright
Ro-Sham-Bo Congo
Top Monkey
Slap Happy
Buzz
PDQ Test
Down By the Banks
Do As I Say
People To People Twister
Touch That
Dog Shake
Eileen
Deportment Tag
Knee Tag
Bill & the Button Factory
Primal Scream

PAIRED SHARES

One of the most potent tools for spicing up any ice-breaker

AT A GLANCE

At appropriate intervals, you ask the members of a pair or small group to share their thoughts on a particular topic.

WHAT YOU NEED
1 - 5 mins

WHAT TO DO

I'm putting this 'ice-breaker' right up front because it can be integrated into any one or all of the remaining activities in this section. When you invite people to share, you build energy, while the process of sharing itself goes a long way toward chipping away at the ice that is often present in groups, especially when they first meet. Like American Express, I never leave a program without using this technique at some point to help me break the ice. Works like a charm.

Pepper your program, especially at the start, with some well-placed pair-shared opportunities. Works best when you have designed lots of mixing and interaction into your program, moving from pairs to threesomes, half-half splits, back to pairs, etc. But, pick your moment – don't bog down every level of interaction as a time to share, or it will get old.

Activities such as Categories (page 45), Spectrums (page 48), and any of the partner activities are ideal for

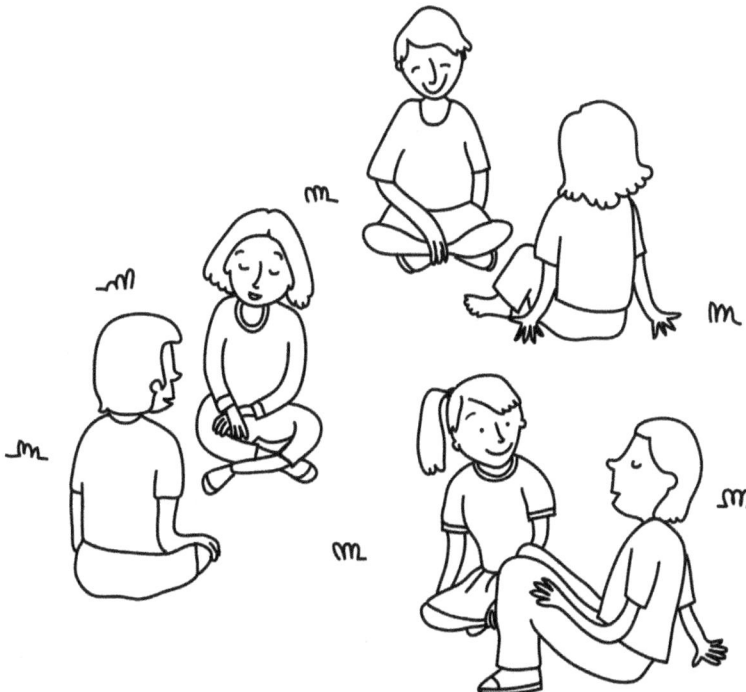

dropping in a couple of paired-shares along the way.

What to share? Sky's the limit. Sometimes, it makes sense to invite conversation around the topic at hand. For example, if you asked your group to split according to who is the eldest, youngest or in-between in their family, invite conversation about the good, the bad and the ugly of this relative status. Or, try some of my favourites below.

Variations

- What did you want to be when you 'grew up'?
- What was your most memorable adventure experience?
- The way I would describe my family is...
- My fondest memories of another person are ...
- What was your most embarrassing moment?
- Describe the most irritating driving habit you see on the roads today.
- What is the one talent or skill you wish you had?
- Describe the naughtiest thing you did as a kid.
- Name one famous person (dead or alive) you would love to have dinner with tonight.
- If you were 20 years old again, and knew what you know now, what would you do differently?
- Name three of your most important values.
- The thing that makes me different from other people is ...
- If you could ask a 'Higher-Being' just one question, what would it be?
- If you could be invisible for just one hour, what would you do?
- Some of the things that make me happy are...
- If you had a tattoo on your body, where would you put it, and what design would it be?
- If you won the lottery, what is the first thing you would do?

CATEGORIES

The perfect ice-breaker – ideal for mixing people in a fun and non-threatening manner

AT A GLANCE

Your group splits into a variety of smaller groupings, according to a series of categories you announce.

WHAT YOU NEED

10 – 20 mins

WHAT TO DO

Ask your group to separate according to the categories or groupings you are about to announce. For example, if the category is "COLOUR OF YOUR PANTS," everyone wearing blue jeans will group together. Sometimes, individuals may find themselves alone, but in most cases, small groupings of commonality will develop. Upon identifying each of the groups, announce the next split. You can keep splitting folks for as long as they are having fun, or you run out of ideas.

For mixing purposes, alternate between two-group splits and multi-group splits. The idea is to invite your group to meet as many new people as possible. To this end, if you have the time and the inclination, as soon as the groups have formed, give the participants a few moments to say hello to one another, or perhaps share something of relevance to the category, e.g., "What was so cool about being the oldest / youngest / in-between child in your family?"

Here are just a few sample and fun group categories. There are simply hundreds of them out there, so please, don't hesitate to make up your own, or tempt them from your group.

Simple half-half splits:

- Arm that ends up crossed over the top of the other, when folded on your chest
- Leg you put into your pants, shorts, underwear, etc. first when dressing
- Preference for cooking or cleaning up
- Preference for washing or drying dishes
- Position of your thumbs, that is left or right on top, when you clasp your hands together so that your fingers interlock
- Last digit of your home telephone number. All the odd numbers – 1, 3, 5, 7 or 9 – get together, and the even numbers do the same.
- When presented with a 'good news / bad news story,' which do you prefer to hear first?

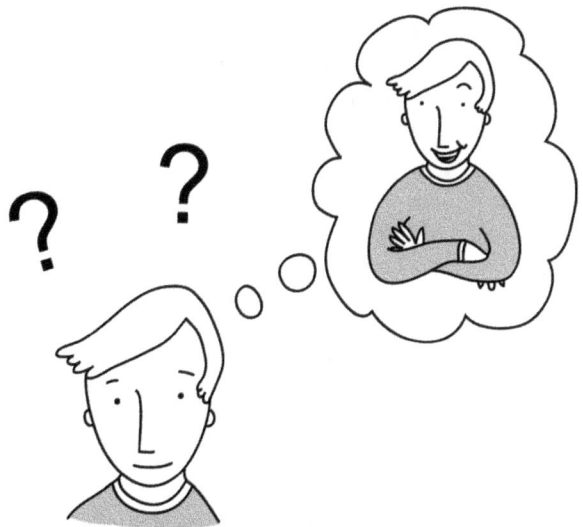

- Preference for the way toilet paper spills off the roll – like a waterfall, over the top and forward, or against the back towards the wall
- Number of street you live at – odds and evens

Simple multi-group splits:

- Month / zodiac sign in which you were born
- Number of continents you have visited
- Number of siblings in your family, including yourself

- Colour of your eyes, hair, socks, etc
- Type of shoes you are wearing (not necessarily their brand)
- Which shoulder(s) you hold a carry-bag – right, left or both shoulders
- How often you shave each week?
- Distance you have travelled to get here (use clumps of distances, such as 0-5 km, 5-10 km, etc. (10 miles, 150 miles, etc)
- Number of items you recycle at home, e.g., plastic, glass, tin, paper, etc.

Variation

Use to divide a large group into roughly random and even teams. If you are looking for an even split, and just don't seem to find a category that fits, simply use the old scientific method of indiscriminately moving a few people ("Hey, you and you, move over here.") to even out the groupings.

VOWEL ORCHESTRA

A choral way to mix your group and form four or five smaller groups

AT A GLANCE

People sing aloud the sound of the first vowel of their name to locate other like-vowelled members and form a group.

WHAT YOU NEED

1 – 2 mins

WHAT TO DO

You could use this simple little activity as another Category (see page 45); however, if you have the time and the inclination, it can take on a life of its own.

Ask everyone to close their eyes, and

to think of the first vowel of their first name. Then, invite them to imagine in their mind's eye the most beautiful voice in the world singing that vowel out loud. Think of the treatment a full-bodied, no-holds-barred opera singer would give that vowel. Now, invite them to open their eyes, and reproduce that magnificent sound as best and as strongly as they can.

After a few tentative starts, you will soon hear a cacophony of "AAA"s, "EEE"s, "III"s and "OOO"s, and if you're lucky a few "UUU"s (there never seem to be many of these). The idea is for each person to keep belting out

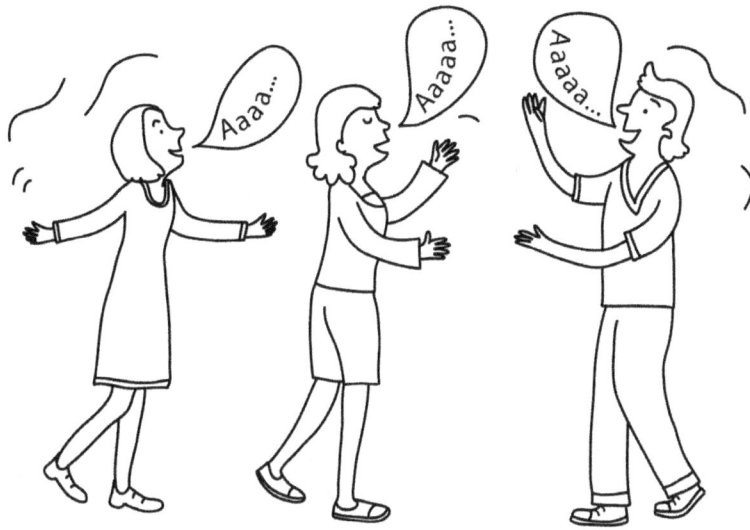

their vowel until they find everyone else who is singing the same sound. Like attracts like.

Now, you could just stop here and move onto whatever activity you planned that required four or five smaller groups. Or, as I would recommend, have some harmonic fun on the way.

Invite each group of vowels (suitably separated from everyone else) to perform, so to speak, a little choral masterpiece. Waving your conductor's baton in the air, tempt each group as you point to them to sing their 'vowel aria' in harmony together. Blend the vowels together, make some short, others long, soft notes and loud notes, whatever. You get the idea. Clearly, the more you put into your role as conductor, the more your group will respond.

This never ceases to inspire a lot of smiles. Often, people who would never consider themselves singers are amazed at how gorgeous their voice sounds when it's mixed with a large group. They probably also think they sound good in the shower!

Variations

- Use the first vowel of a person's last name. This way, you have a better chance of getting closer to five small groups that are more or less even in number.

- For a more complex version, ask people to sing the sound of the initial of their first name. This of course will include all of the consonants, attracting all sounds of a similar harmony (you know, the last part of the sound). For example, everyone whose name starts with a D, P or T will associate with the EEEs.

JELLY BEAN TRADE

A fast and delicious mixer for sweet-tooths

AT A GLANCE
  Starting with 10 random jelly beans, each person trades beans with other group members to be the first to collect 10 of the same colour.

WHAT YOU NEED
  At least 10 jelly beans per person
  Paper bags or other receptacle (if you wish to avoid as much of the sticky as possible)
  5 mins

WHAT TO DO
  Everyone starts with 10 randomly picked jelly beans, or other variously coloured, sweet treats. On your signal, everyone is asked to mix with all others and start trading – one for one – so that at the end of the exercise, you are left with 10 jelly beans of the same colour. The first to achieve this goal wins.
  Well, actually everyone wins, because whether you are first or last, you should still have 10 treats in your hand – no matter what colour. And what better way to celebrate than to eat them! OK, so who has a black jelly bean to trade?

Variations

- Go backwards. Start with a set of treats the same colour. Your goal is to collect all the different colours.

- Not as tasty, but try different coloured pieces of paper.

SPECTRUMS

A passive 'get to know you better' game

AT A GLANCE
  People respond to a series of questions by standing between two imaginary points of a spectrum.

WHAT YOU NEED
  10 - 15 mins

WHAT TO DO
  Create in the mind's eye of your group the concept of an imaginary line that stretches between two points – be it two walls, a couple of trees, whatever. Describe this space as a spectrum, suggesting that if black was at one end and white the other, all the shades of grey would be in between. Having created this metaphor, announce to your group that you would like each individual to place him or herself along this spectrum according to their responses to a series of questions and scenarios. They can choose to be anywhere along the imaginary line, but stress that it is their decision, and they should try to not be influenced by where their peers and / or friends are standing.

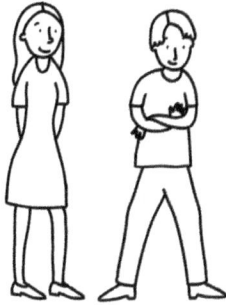 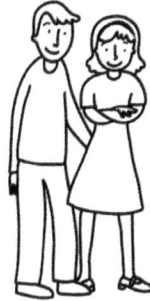 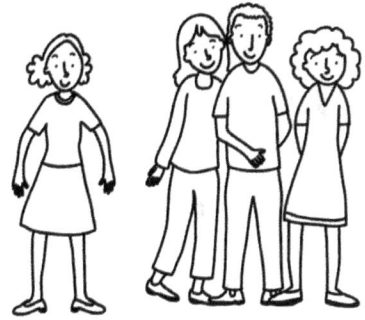

black ....white

For example, explain that the spectrum represents how we, as individuals, typically view waking up in the morning. On the left-hand side of the spectrum, we have the early risers, those folks who just can't wait to get out of bed, and are pumped as soon as their feet hit the floor. Then, at the extreme right-hand side, we have those poor souls who hit the snooze button twice and need three cups of coffee to remember even what day it is. And of course, everyone else fits somewhere in between.

Upon announcing each scenario or question, ask people to move to where they belong within the spectrum. There are no right or wrong answers. But the depth and breadth of the spread will reflect a number of characteristics about the group. From time to time, invite the group to observe where they are generally situated, and perhaps even ask them to share with a few neighbours or with the larger group what this might mean. Or, of course, you could simply move people from one spectrum to the next solely for the purposes of mixing, getting to know one another and having fun.

Here are a few spectrums to start with, then make up a few of your own.

- Your exercise regime – never to several hours a day
- Job preference – totally indoors to totally outdoors
- Car security – never lock your car to always lock your car, even if you are gone for 30 seconds.
- Preferred home – deep inner-city to remote wilderness
- Preferred landscape – mountains to sea
- Time of year born – January to December
- Favourite sport – A to Z

Variation

Use this technique to process or debrief a group experience, for example, create a spectrum of "How well the group communicated" where one end is woeful and the other is without fault.

MAPPING

A simple spatial exercise that will quickly invite your group to mix

AT A GLANCE

In response to a series of statements, people move themselves to a position relative to a centre point – representing their current location – which maps their place in an imaginary world.

WHAT YOU NEED

Any object to mark the centre of your space

5 – 10 mins

WHAT TO DO

Place an object, such as a witch's hat or cone, in the centre of your space, and ask your group to bunch on in around it. Explain that this object represents where you and your group are standing right now, and happens to also represent the centre of a giant map of the world, which is framed by the boundaries of your room, playing space, etc. It's often useful to point out where north, south, east and west are too just so people can get their bearings.

Basically, you're asking people to imagine that they are standing in the middle of a huge imaginary map of the world. Your next instruction is to explain that you will call out a series of statements or questions, and would like each person to move from their current position to a spot on the map that best represents their response.

It is common for some people to orient themselves near, if not, right on top of other people. That's OK. In fact, I would suggest that's a great opportunity to invite some sharing.

Here's a series of questions I have often used to get to know my group a little more:

- Where in the world were you born?
- Where in the world would you love to go on holiday?

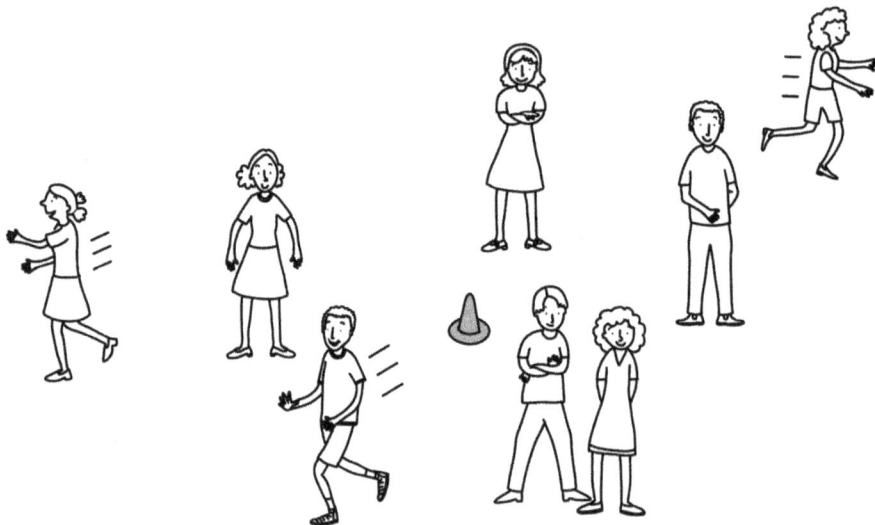

- If you could live somewhere else in the world for a year, where would you go?
- Move to a country that speaks one of your favourite foreign languages.
- Which continent would you most like to visit?

- Move to the country that is renowned for producing your favourite cuisine.
- Where is the one place on earth you would not want to visit?
- Move to the location of your most memorable adventure experience.

Variations

- Create an image of your playing space being your local community or town only. Ask a series of questions that relate to local events, pastimes, histories, etc.
- Develop a meaningful metaphor in which your map and questions relate directly to a particular subject or course of study. For example, health and wellness, international relations and culture.

SIGNATURE BINGO

An active mixer that's all about fishing for information about people

AT A GLANCE

People aim to get as many signatures on their bingo sheet as possible by seeking other group members who match certain criteria.

WHAT YOU NEED

Sheet of paper per person, each marked with a large square with rows and columns

A pen for everyone

10 – 20 mins

WHAT TO DO

First, you need to prepare a sheet of paper marked to look a bit like a BINGO sheet, you know, 5 rows by 5 columns = 25 squares. Make it 6 x 6 or 7 x 7 if you have a really large group. If in doubt, always go large. Make a copy for each person.

Fill each square with a short instruction, such as "Ask someone who was born in February to sign here." Variety is the key, and don't make the criteria too obvious so that a simple observation will suffice, e.g., "Find someone who has red hair." Mixing and signing is good, but encouraging people to talk with one another is better.

Here's a short list of possible signature criteria.

Ask someone who rode the bus to school to sign here.

... was born overseas

... has seven letters in their first name

... is taller than you

... has the same number of siblings as you

... owns a dog at home

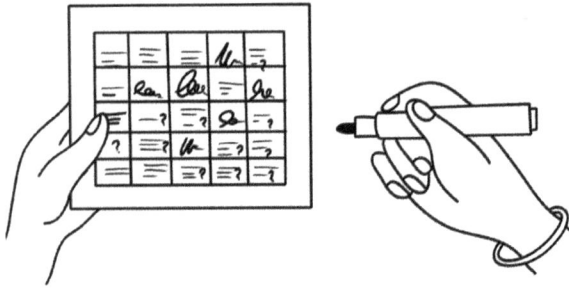

... has travelled interstate for their holidays

... likes cereal for breakfast

... knows how to waltz

... is the same age as you.

You can probably guess the next bit. Each person frantically seeks as many people in the group to sign their sheet, i.e., when a person matching the criteria is found, they are asked to sign the relevant square. The aim? To be the first person to obtain five signatures in a row (up, down or diagonal), or the first to fill the entire sheet, or as many squares as possible in the allotted time. Maybe they get a prize at the end, or maybe they don't.

Unlike regular bingo, it's not necessary to make each sheet unique. However, there should be many more people than there are bingo squares to provide ample opportunities for mixing.

If you (or the group) know each other very well, create questions that feature at least one really unique attribute about each individual. Such as "Find the person who has been hit by lightning twice," or "Ask someone to recite the alphabet using sign language."

Variations

- Create a BINGO sheet full of numbers, where the numbers represent anything related to another person. For example, a "13" could represent one person's age, "4" could be the number of siblings in someone's family or "23" could be the street address of another. Add the relevant criteria to the signature in the box.

- As above, but this time the numbers represent birth dates, i.e., cover numbers 1 to 31.

- Make the criteria in each square active. Thinking out loud, here's a short list of possible actions:

  – Ask someone to do five push-ups.
  – Ask a male to sing "Jingle Bells."
  – Ask a female to recite a nursery rhyme.
  – Using your non-dominant hand, shake hands with someone you don't know.
  – Leap frog over someone three times.
  – Whisper your name into the ear of someone taller than you.
  – Ask someone to teach you a dance step.
  – Find someone who is left-handed to sign your sheet.
  – Ask someone to say "Unique New York" five times quickly.
  – Find someone who is having a birthday this month and sing "Happy Birthday" to them.

NONSENSE NUMBERS

A really fun way to learn a lot about a small group in a short space of time

AT A GLANCE

Small groups attempt to record the highest number of points possible by adding a set of pre-determined numbers based on specific and diverse attributes of its members.

WHAT YOU NEED

One sheet of 'Nonsense Numbers' instructions per small group

A pen for each group

10 – 20 mins

WHAT TO DO

Your first step is to prepare your Nonsense Numbers sheet in advance. It will consist of a series of questions that can all be answered with a set of numbers, which are then added together to give one total. For example, one question may ask every person to count the number of letters that spell their name. Mine would be 4 (Mark) plus 4 (Alan) plus 7 (Collard) to equal 15 points. This is added to the sum of the score of my colleagues.

I have prepared a generic Nonsense Numbers sheet in the Activity Supplement on page 231 to get you started, but feel free to create your own criteria – there is no magic here.

Here's how it works. Divide into smaller groups. Hand each group a copy of your 'Nonsense Numbers' sheet with a pen or two. Explain that you would like each group to calculate the numerical value for each category by sharing the relevant information about one other.

Your instructions will prescribe how many points a group will score for particular attributes or experiences. For a bit of fun, and to flush out those really interesting tid-bits of information about your group, offer bonus points to reward particularly unique characteristics. Add all the numbers, and you get a GIQ (Group Identity Quotient) for each group. Highest score wins – whatever that means.

Set a time limit if you like, but it's not often necessary. The data is so nonsensical, the criteria seems to drive the group forward anyway.

Variations

- Design a set of criteria that relates to a specific field or realm, e.g., profession or school-based attributes. For example, if you are working with a group of teachers, you could specify the following criteria:

  - 1 pt for each separate grade taught, and 5 pts for teaching six or more grades

  - 1 pt for each state in which they have taught, and 5 pts for teaching overseas; etc.

VORTEX

Classic way to mix and get to know people in a structured manner

AT A GLANCE

People form two circles, one inside and facing the other, and speak with a sequence of partners about a series of topics suggested by the leader.

WHAT YOU NEED

Seats for everyone (optional)
10 – 15 mins

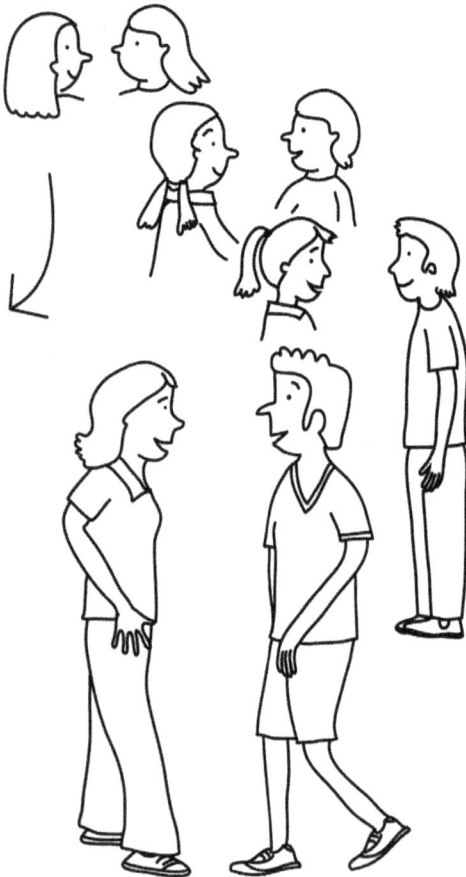

WHAT TO DO

Often, I find the instruction of "Set up two circles, one inside the other," the hardest part of any exercise. So, my next instructions represent the most successful method I have found to get it right the first time.

Ask everyone to find a partner who has similar length of hair (or other favourite random-splitting assignment). In pairs, one person agrees to become '1,' the other '2.' Are you still with me? Now, invite all of the '1's to form a large circle facing inwards. Once assembled, you invite all of the '2's to step inside the circle, locate and face their partners. You should now have two equally portioned circles, each facing the other. Phew.

With everyone looking at you in eager anticipation of what's next, you give your first question. See Paired Shares (page 43) for some fantastic suggestions. Allow each partnership to chat away for a minute or two, and then upon getting everyone's attention again, explain the process of change. By this, you will ask one circle at a time to move to their left or right as many people as you nominate to face a new partner. For example, "NUMBER '1's, MOVE THREE PEOPLE TO YOUR RIGHT."

Invite newly facing partners to introduce themselves for a moment, and then launch into your next probing getting-to-know-you question. Continue until energy starts to ebb.

Variations

- To mix it up even more, ask everyone who is wearing a particular coloured garment, say red, to swap spots with their partners. This will mix some of the '1's with the '2's, providing a chance for some '1's to meet a '1', and vice versa.

- Invite questions from the floor.

MINTIE GAME

An awesome mixer that is as effective as it is delicious

AT A GLANCE
Starting with 10 treats each, people aim to earn more treats by causing as many people as possible to say the word "YES" in their ensuing conversations.

WHAT YOU NEED
10 'Minties' or other sweet treats (preferably wrapped), per person
5 - 10 mins

WHAT TO DO
Ohhhh, this seems so easy to do, but I swear the simple exercise of not saying "YES" is so hard.

I first played this game with 'Minties' (refreshingly chewy mint lolly), but it works just as well with any sweet treat. Distribute an exact number, say 10, to everyone in your group, and then just as quickly, tell them not to eat them – just yet!

Now, invite your group to mix and mingle with each other, engaging in conversation as often as possible. Encourage them to introduce themselves, exchange pleasantries etc, etc, and then engage in the fine art of conversation. But this is not just any form of conversation; your goal is to cause the other to say the word "YES." Every time your partner utters this pleasantly uncomplicated word, you gain a Mintie. The person with the most Minties at the end 'wins.'

My favourite line to gain a quick Mintie? I spy anyone on their own, approach them and calmly ask "Do you have any Minties left? "Yes I do, er... arghhhhhh.." Works like a charm.

Variation

Substitute the word "YES" with other colloquially popular words such as "LIKE," and if you want to make it really difficult – the word "AND." It's near impossible!

WHO AM I?

A great mixer that will have your group guessing who they are

AT A GLANCE

With the name of a 'celebrity' stuck to their back, an individual will attempt to identify who the celebrity is by asking other group members a series of Yes / No questions about this person.

WHAT YOU NEED

A 'celebrity' index card for each person
Sticky tape
10 – 20 mins

WHAT TO DO

Your first step is to create a set of index cards with the names of famous, well-known, celebrity type people written on them. Ideally, use a different 'celebrity' for each member of your group. For example, Mickey Mouse, Brad Pitt, Nicole Kidman, Steve Irwin, Michael Jordan, Princess Diana, Michael Jackson, and so on. Throw in a few lesser-known, obscure celebrities to mix it up a bit too.

Gather your group, and randomly, yet secretly, stick an index card on the back of each person. It's OK for others to see it, as long as the person to whom it belongs does not. Next, explain that each person's mission is to identify 'who they are' by asking other members of the group as few Yes / No questions as possible. That is, a person is only permitted to ask a question that can be answered "YES" or "NO."

It works like this. On "GO," everyone seeks a partner. After exchanging pleasantries (including their real names), each person will ask one Yes / No question of their partner. Having already peeked at their partner's 'celebrity' status, the other person will answer "YES" or "NO." Nothing else, no hints, no miming, nothing. If the person being asked is not sure, rather than say "MAYBE," they should ask their partner to ask a new question.

The first question might be, "AM I MALE?" Their partner responds with a "YES" or "NO," and then follows with their question, perhaps "AM I AN ANIMAL?" To encourage lots of interaction, instruct your group to ask only one question of one person, before moving on to someone new.

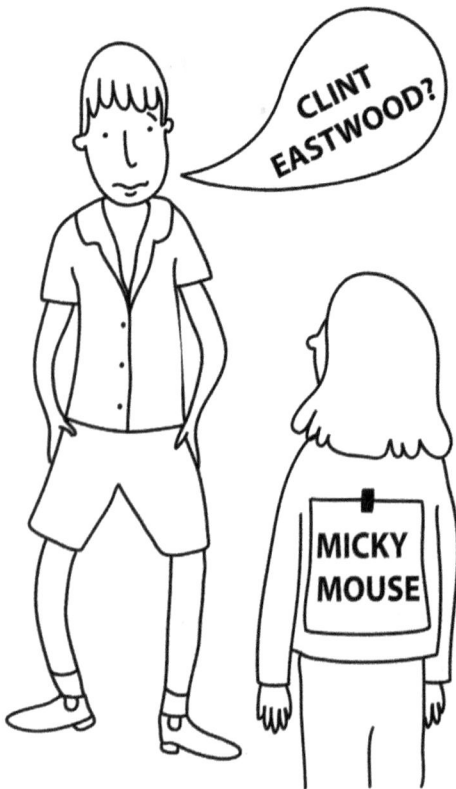

Truth is always obvious to those who know it, so it's wonderful watching the frustration of a 'celebrity' try to work out who they are. Keep the interaction flowing, until everyone has guessed their identity.

Variations

- Allow the 'celebrity' to continue asking questions until they receive a "NO" from their partner, at which point, they must move on to a new person.

- For groups who know each other well, write the names of group members on the cards.

- For less interaction, but tons of fun, invite several volunteers to sit in front of your group, and stick an index card (with a celebrity's name on it) on each of their foreheads, i.e., so everyone other than the volunteers, can see who they are. See Celebrity Head on page 195 for full description.

ACRONYMS

I've found this to be the most successful arrival activity yet

AT A GLANCE

A group attempts to decipher a variety of acronyms as they are presented one after another.

WHAT YOU NEED

List of 'acronyms' printed on index cards or sheets of paper
Paper and pens (optional)
10 – 20 mins

WHAT TO DO

You know how it feels when the clock says it's time to start, but it's obvious that not everyone is here. I hate waiting, so I have developed a bunch of really simple, non-threatening activities that can occupy (think reward) those folks who are on time, yet not disrupt the group's fun when the late-comers finally appear.

Well in advance, grab a magazine, newspaper or both and start flicking through the pages spotting as many acronyms (you know, a word that is formed from the initials of other words) as you can. I'm sure you know many off the top of your head. Write these 'words' onto a set of index cards or sheets of paper. You'll need at least 40 or more.

Can't think of any, here's a start (answers on page 232):

PIN	DOA	QANTAS	LASER	NATO	AD
ANZAC	FAQ	BBC	BMW	LED	HMS
RAM	FUBAR	NIMBY	ATM	SCUBA	pH
MGM	WHO	FUNN	UFO	DINK	RSVP
MASH	GSOH	CEO	UNESCO	ISBN	IVF

The basic idea is to present this series of cards, turning one card over at a time, asking your group to decipher as many of the acronyms as they can, in as little time as possible. Get it right (bing!) and you show the next card. Can't work it out, either tell them the answer, or put the card aside to work on later as you move onto the next one.

As an opening (arrival) activity, let me describe my all-time favourite version. I make an 'unofficial' start by asking people to bunch on in, sit them down (often on the floor), introduce myself briefly and pull out the cards. Within a few minutes and a dozen or so cards, I have not only fostered engagement and some laughter (I often encourage silly answers), but also introduced many elements of the program (by deliberately placing certain cards within the pile). For example, I'll add acronyms such as FUNN, CBC and FUBAR into the sequence and make a quick comment about their relevance to my program before I move onto the next card. I've found this to be an awesome, creative way to kick off many programs.

Really large group? I find that the business-card-sized acronyms are good for up to forty or so people. Yes, the cards are small, but it encourages people to move in. Beyond this number, I graduate to large-index-card-sized acronyms. More than 70, try writing the acronyms on a whiteboard, or holding up printed signs.

For other great arrival activities, see Wordles on page 59 and Alphabet Equations on page 60.

Hey, did you know that ACRONYM is really an acronym? A Contrived Reduction Of Nomenclature Yielding Mnemonics! Or, how about Annoyingly Cryptic References Of Names You Make-up?

Variations

- Separate into smaller groups, and hand each a number of acronym cards. Their object is to correctly guess as many as possible, perhaps within a time limit.

- As above, but this time add a number of blank index cards and supply a magazine or newspaper. Each small group is now challenged to find a variety of acronyms within the pages, write them on the blank cards, and invite another group to translate as many as possible.

- As above, and if you feel the group will act appropriately, ask each small group to invent as many made-up, zany acronyms (using real or nonsensical words) as they can in two minutes, e.g., YAHOO is Young At Heart Or Older. You could even ask them to challenge another group to guess the answers. When kept above the belt, totally hilarious.

WORDLES

Fun, cryptic and awfully infectious brainteasers that stimulate lateral thinking

AT A GLANCE

Small groups attempt to decipher a series of cryptic puzzles consisting of words and patterns.

WHAT YOU NEED

Series of 'Wordles' printed on index cards or sheets of paper

Paper and pens (if you want the answers recorded)

10 – 20 mins

WHAT TO DO

First of all, you need to prepare a set of 'Wordle' (WORD puzzLE) cards in advance. I have provided a bunch of my favourites in the Activity Supplement on page 233, but here's three to whet your appetite.

The object is to invite your group to decipher the hidden word or phrase as quickly as possible, or simply to reward creativity. It's a good idea to decipher a sample Wordle up front to establish the type of 'lateral' thinking required. For example, the first Wordle is "Hole in One," i.e., the word HOLE is situated in the middle of the word ONE. The other two are "Feeling Under The Weather" and "Robin Hood" If measuring success is necessary, ask your group to solve as many Wordles within a prescribed time limit.

Personally, I love using this exercise either as an arrival activity, or to stimulate creative thinking and brainstorming before a complex problem-solving activity.

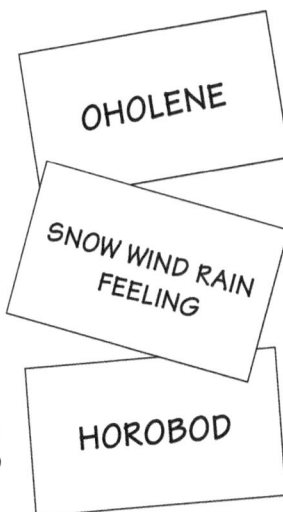

OHOLENE

SNOW WIND RAIN FEELING

HOROBOD

Variations

- As an arrival activity, assemble your group in front of a stack of face-down Wordle cards, and turn one card over at a time, asking the group to figure out its meaning before turning to the next one.

- Separate into small groups, and supply each with a set of 10 Wordle cards face down. One card is turned over at a time, and as soon as the Wordle is deciphered, the group can turn over the next card. I recommend that the group stay with a card for no longer than two minutes, at which point they can put that card to the side (to keep working on it), and turn over a fresh card.

- Stick a series of Wordle cards on the walls of your room (or hall, trees, etc), and invite your group – either as individuals or small groups – to brood over the cards in any order they choose. Great for mixing and building energy, and for really large groups.

- Give a set of blank cards to your small groups, and ask them to invent their own set of Wordles.

ALPHABET EQUATIONS

Another great puzzler that stimulates creative thought

AT A GLANCE

A group attempts to decipher a series of puzzles by substituting an array of related initials for the words of a common phrase.

WHAT YOU NEED

List of 'Alphabet Equations' printed on index cards or sheets of paper.
Paper and pens (optional)
10 – 20 mins

WHAT TO DO

Used as an activity in its own right, or designed as a beaut arrival activity, present this activity much like you would Wordles or Acronyms. In this case, your group needs to identify what the capitalised letters in each of a series of 'equations' represents. For example 26 = L of the A represents 26 Letters of the Alphabet.

Using this as an arrival activity, I often assemble my group in front of a stack of face-down equations, and turn one card over at a time, asking the group to figure out the phrase before turning to the next one.

I'll start you off with a set of Alphabet Equations below (see page 235 for the answers), but there are tons of other phrases you could use to form an equation.

7	=	W of the AW
1001	=	AN
12	=	S of the Z
54	=	C in a P with Js
88	=	PK
13	=	S on the AF
32	=	DF at which WF
18	=	H on a GC
57	=	HV
66	=	B in the B
50	=	S in the U
14	=	D in a F
21	=	D on a D
3	=	S and you're O
6	=	S on a H
4	=	Q in a G
90	=	D in a RA
29	=	D in F in a LY
64	=	S on a CB

Variations

- Divide into small groups, and supply each with a set of 10 equation cards face down. One card is turned over at a time, and as soon as the equation is solved, the group can turn over the next card. I recommend that the group stays with a card for no longer then two minutes, at which point they can put that card to the side (to keep working on it), and then turn over a fresh card.

- Stick a series of alphabet equation cards on the walls of your room (or hall, trees, etc), and invite your group – either as individuals or small groups – to brood over the cards in any order they choose. Great for mixing and building energy, and for really large groups.

- Give a set of blank cards to your small groups, and ask them to invent their own set of Alphabet Equations.

COMFORT CIRCLE

Fantastic way to prepare your group for an adventure of sorts

AT A GLANCE

Individuals position themselves in relation to two concentric circles representing the varying degrees of challenge they perceive in response to a series of 'adventure' statements.

WHAT YOU NEED

Two longish ropes 1 x 8 metre (26') and 1 x 16 metre (52')

10 – 15 mins

WHAT TO DO

Are you looking for a perfect way to prepare your group for an upcoming adventure, or perhaps to help broaden their understanding of what challenge is? Look no further.

Set up an area where you can establish two concentric circles (one inside the other) – the smaller one being about 2 – 3 metres (7 – 10') diameter, the second about 4 – 5 metres (14 – 17') diameter.

Start with your group standing around the outside of the largest circle looking in. Next, you want to generate the notion that what your group is looking at represents a scale that measures the level of comfort or challenge that may be perceived in any given activity or experience. Kick off describing the smallest circle in more detail, and then work your way out. Use your own words and examples, but it goes something like this:

Inside Circle – Comfort Zone:

Everything you know and have learned is found within this circle / area. And because you know it or have learned it, you are comfortable with it, so there is little if any stress involved. For example, I am comfortable speaking the English language. Driving a motor vehicle also rests within my comfort zone.

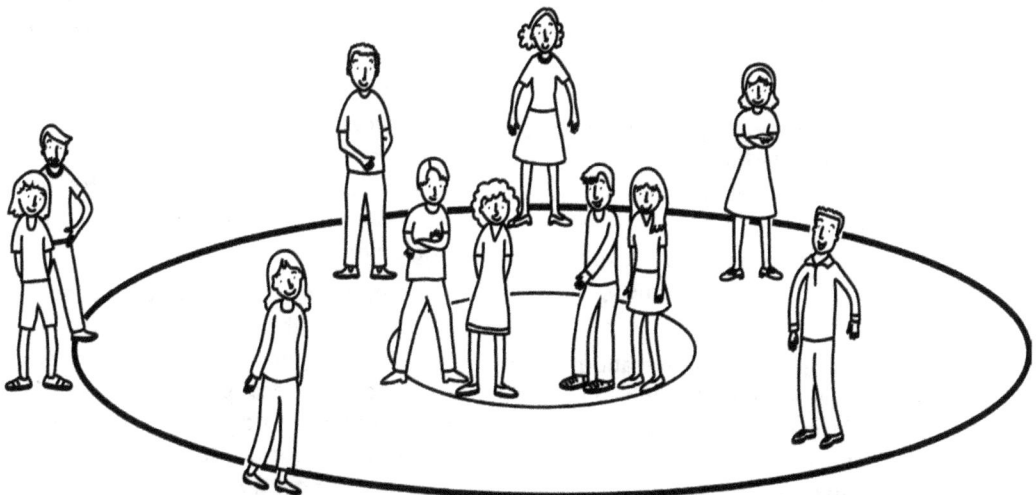

Larger Circle – Stretch Zone:

This is where all meaningful learning occurs. When we step outside of our comfort zone, our abilities, knowledge and expertise are stretched. The more we enter our stretch zones, the more comfortable we become, thereby allowing our comfort zone to grow. This is the primary aim of all education, to grow people's comfort zone, by inviting them into the stretch zone. For example, I was in my stretch zone when I first started to rock-climb.

Beyond the Large Circle – Panic Zone:

Also known as the 'fight or flight' zone. When people find themselves inside this zone of 'comfort,' it's all about survival. It is rare for anyone to learn anything within this zone, other than not to let it happen again. This is where people are pushed beyond their limits, and retreat promising never to return. Examples of panic may include swimming with sharks and jumping out of planes.

OK, you've set the scene, now for the fun part. Explain that you will now invite your group to consider a series of hypothetical situations, and will ask them to physically place themselves (stand) in relation to the degree to which they would be comfortable. I always start off with a few scenarios, and then hand over to the group for their ideas. Here are some wonderful openers:

- You spot a big snake about to slither its way through the middle of the group. Where would you be – within your comfort, stretch or panic zone?

- A friend has asked you to go bungy-jumping…
- You've finally decided to ask the cutest, most popular girl / boy in the class for a date…
- After two months of dating, you are about to meet the parents for the first time…
- After a long silence, you finally decide to call everyone's attention and explain that you disagree with what's happening in the group…
- You have suddenly been asked to give a 30 minute speech to an audience of 300 people in 2 hours about a topic you know little about…
- You have to sing a song in front of a group of your peers unaccompanied…

Be sure to present or encourage a good mix of adventures, reflecting mental, physical and emotional risks / challenges. Also, it works best when individuals are not overly influenced by where others position themselves. To this end, carefully consider your preparation (i.e., can people make safe decisions?) before introducing this exercise.

After ten or so minutes, pause the group for a moment, and ask them to review what's just transpired. Discussion in response to the following questions can be a really powerful way to groom a safe and supportive learning environment:

- What did you observe about the group as the activity progressed?
- What might these observations say about our group?
- What impact does this knowledge have on our group as we embark on our next adventure?

Variation

Present the zones with an X and Y axis, where X represents the level of perceived challenge (comfort, stretch, panic), and Y represents the degree of actual risk present (none to lots). For example, spotting a big snake may make most people move into right-hand side of the X axis (high perceived risk), but if it wasn't venomous (low actual risk), some may position themselves lower on the Y scale.

SIT DOWN IF...

A fun get-to-know-my-group better activity

AT A GLANCE
Standing to begin, people sit down when they hear a statement or category that applies to them, all the time hoping to be one of the few people left standing at the end.

WHAT YOU NEED
Set of statements prepared in advance
5 - 10 mins

WHAT TO DO
With your group standing in front of their chairs, or simply in an open space, explain that you are about to announce a series of statements that may or may not apply to each person. The idea is that for every statement that does apply to an individual, that person is asked to sit down. Sometimes lots of people will find their seat, other times, only one or two will need to. As you will read from my examples, there are times when nobody will dare take their seat for fear of embarrassment!
You continue to read from your list of statements, until you have either exhausted your group, or there are only a couple of people remaining.
Here's a sample list of statements, in no particular order:

Sit down if you...

• Didn't apply deodorant today
• Are wearing at least one sock with a hole in it
• Drive a Volkswagen

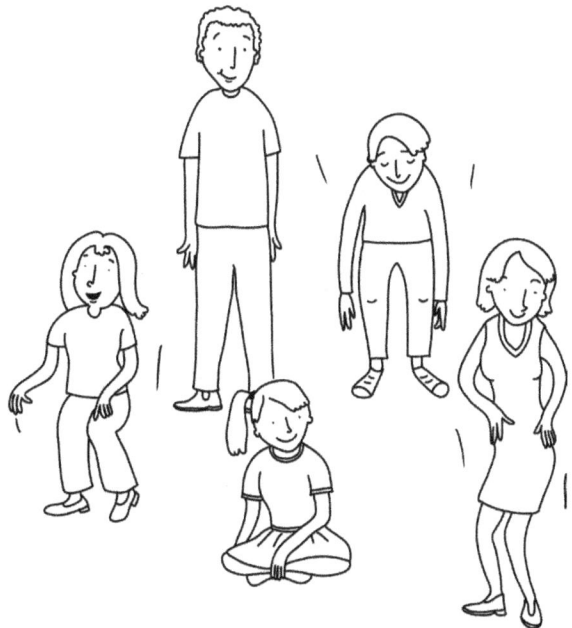

- Sing in the shower
- Have shaved today
- Are mad at someone
- Believe that two people on a date should share expenses
- Are ticklish
- Weigh less than 50 kg (110 lbs)
- Own more than two telephones (including mobiles)
- Have eaten a snail
- Have never lied to your mother

- Received a traffic infringement notice in the past year
- Have a false tooth
- Have an 'outie' belly-button
- Are in love

As you can tell, these are not your common, garden-variety types of getting-to-know-you questions. Mix them up, throw in some fun ones, some revealing ones and above all, some quirky ones.

Variations

- Develop a set of statements or categories that apply to a defined area, such as school, work or a particular field of study.

- Introduce the rule that anyone who sits down in the first two rounds is entitled to stand back up again if a later statement or question applies to them. They of course must sit down on the next one that applies to them, as per usual.

ALL MY NEIGHBOURS

A 'get-to-know-you-better' game with a difference

AT A GLANCE

Starting from a seated position, individuals move to their left around the circle in response to a series of questions posed by the group.

WHAT YOU NEED

A chair for everyone

10 – 20 mins

WHAT TO DO

This activity is best suited to a group that is already comfortable with one another.

The basic set-up is a circle of people, everyone sitting on a chair facing inwards. Explain to your group that each person's mission is to move around the circle, one seat at a time, and return to the seat they started in. Depending on how many people you are working with, this may take a while, or not. But, the 'getting there' is not often the point, right?

Next, describe that to move into the neighbouring seat, each person must be able to answer "YES" to a question that is posed by another member of the group. After a few sample questions from you, invite your group to volunteer the remaining questions.

To illustrate, if the question is "DID YOU BRUSH YOUR TEETH AFTER BREAKFAST THIS MORNING?," everyone

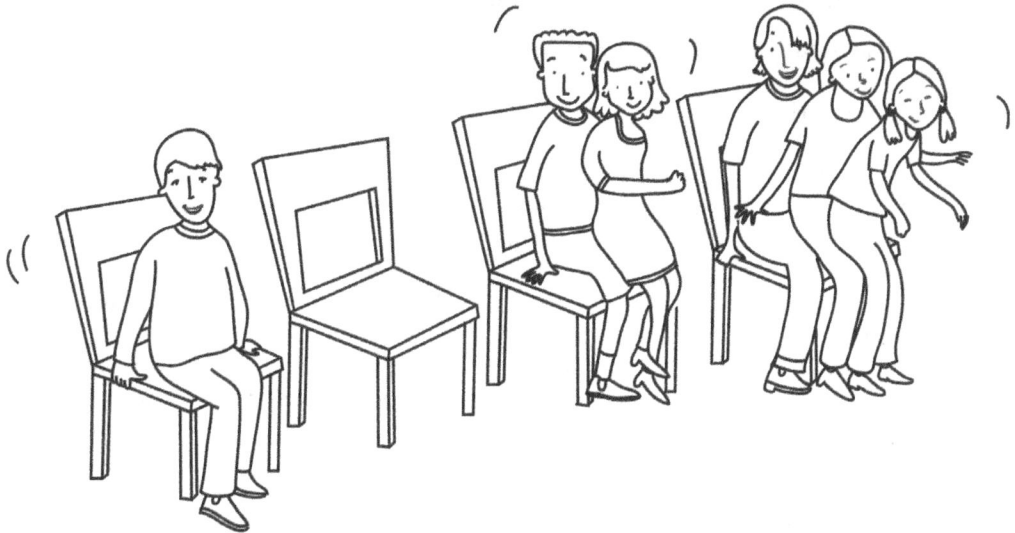

who brushed is entitled to move into the seat on their left. However, it is possible that not everyone brushed their teeth this morning (tsk, tsk), so not every seat will become vacant. Herein lies the fun of the exercise – people are permitted to sit on the laps of others.

After several minutes of questions, it is highly likely that there will be multiple stacks of people sitting on laps identified as belonging to a single chair. Being mindful of the person on the bottom, suggest that after the third companion has landed, all other 'guests' simply stand in front of the chair they belong to.

One final, very important note.

Whenever a person needs to move into a new seat, anyone and everyone who is sitting on their lap or 'higher' must accompany them, whether the question applies to these others or not. For example, imagine that Neil is sitting on Tanya, who sitting on Ingrid, who is seated on the chair. If Tanya is the only one of these three people who has to move, Ingrid will remain on her seat, but Neil will have to follow Tanya to the seat next door. Get it?

Expect a lot of laughter, and lots of clever questions that purposefully dilute or concentrate the traffic jams. Continue until someone returns 'home' or you're exhausted.

Variations

- As a question is called, the questioner can nominate how many spots a person may move.

- Everyone moves on every question. If a person's response is "YES," they move to their left, otherwise they move to their right. Utter chaos, but tons of fun.

DO YOU LOVE YOUR NEIGHBOURS?

A fun getting-to-know-you version of 'Have You Ever?'

AT A GLANCE

One person, standing in the middle of a circle, will ask someone a question, to which the latter will respond with "NO" – to cause his or her neighbours to quickly move positions – or "YES" – to cause everyone else in the circle who relates to a nominated condition to move.

WHAT YOU NEED

A seat for everyone, or spots to mark where each person stands

10 -15 mins

WHAT TO DO

This activity works just as well standing up as is it does sitting down, so it's up to you. If you or your group are pooped, find a seat. Otherwise, distribute enough spot markers, carpet squares, etc for your group to have one each, or in their absence, ask each person to take one shoe off and place it on the floor to mark their spot in the circle.

One person (let's call them the Asker) starts in the middle (without a seat or spot) and approaches a random person in the circle to ask a simple question "DO YOU LOVE YOUR NEIGHBOURS?" Often, after exchanging dodgy glances to their left and right, this person (let's call them the Responder) will respond in one of two ways.

If they say "NO," the two people directly next to them, i.e., the neighbours, automatically jump out of their seats and attempt to swap positions. The fun part is, the Asker is also trying to snatch a seat. Three doesn't go into two empty seats, so one of them ends up 'in the middle' to ask the next question.

However, if the Responder says "YES," they must immediately state a particular qualifying condition such as "I LOVE PEOPLE WITH BLUE EYES." Anyone who matches this description – and this will include the subject's two neighbours if they qualify – are invited to leave the safety of their spot in the circle, and find another. Again, the Asker is seeking to nab a seat too. Note, the qualifying condition does not have to apply to the subject's neighbours – it's just something the Responder makes up to move the group about.

The thrill of anticipating a "YES" or "NO" answer tends to keep people on the edge of their seats, ready to 'snap-into-action' and create a frenzy of traffic inside the circle. So, it's often useful to remind your group to be conscious of other people also shopping frantically for empty seats.

Variations

- When the Responder says "NO," he or she will also call the names of any two people in the circle. These two people and the Responder's two neighbours must vacate their seat and find a new one.
- Invite the two neighbours to both the left and right of the Responder (making four people in total) to move positions. Ensure that anyone seated to the left of the subject, moves to the right, and vice versa.
- If you consider the "Do you love your neighbours?" question a little heavy for your group, try any question that can be answered with a YES or NO answer. For example, "DO YOU LOVE MATHEMATICS?"
- Introduce the rule that for "YES" the Responder will state a condition or description that must apply to at least one of his or her neighbours. This is an awesome exercise for groups who already know each other a little.

FIVE CLUES

Simple guess-the-identity game, with tons of variations

AT A GLANCE

Participants write five 'clues' about their identity onto a card, which is then randomly selected from a pile of cards and read out loud, in order for the rest of the group to guess who the person is.

WHAT YOU NEED

Index card (or sheet of paper) for each player
Pens
10 – 20 mins

WHAT TO DO

This activity works as a name-game for newly-formed groups as well as a great 'get-to-know-you-better' activity for groups who have known each other for a while.

Use a random group-splitting method to divide your group into even teams of at least 10 to 15 people. Give each person a blank index card (or piece of paper) and then instruct them to secretly write five little-known facts or clues about themselves. Allow a couple of minutes to provide an opportunity for the more-inventive in your group to think. They finish off by writing their name at the bottom of the card. A card may read, for example, I HAVE A PET SNAKE; MY MIDDLE NAME IS JULIO; I WAS BORN IN CINCINNATI; I HATE PIZZA; AND THE CARPET IN MY BEDROOM IS GREEN; and then the person's name.

OK, collect all the cards, shuffle those belonging to each team, and you are ready to play.

The object is to challenge a particular group to identify and name the person on the card that you have drawn from the pile (from the other team's stack of cards) in as few clues as possible. That's the key – the group has to guess the person in as few clues as possible. It's fun just watching a group struggle to identify the mystery person as you progress through the clues. Or, you can build the excitement by awarding a diminishing number of points to the guessing team as each clue is read out, for example, five points if they guess on the first clue, four points on the second clue, and so on.

Encourage people to 'think outside the square' as they develop their clues, you know, the sort of clues that most people would never associate with them. Also, it is best for you as the teacher / facilitator to read the cards (rather than invite the guessing team to read the card themselves), to avoid the possibility that a person's handwriting could 'give them away.'

Got a really large group? Split them into teams of six to eight people, read all five clues of say ten to fifteen cards, and challenge each team to identify and name as many of the mystery people as possible.

Variations

- Same as above, but this time instruct each person to add a 'lie' to their set of clues, i.e., each person writes four truths and one lie (something that they have made-up). Now, all five clues are read out as a set, and the guessing team is challenged to identify who the mystery person is in the other team, and to nominate which clue is the lie.

- If you have developed a high level of trust and safety within your group, make it just one clue. Each person writes only one statement, describing an experience that was particularly embarrassing for them.

CATEGORIES WITH A TWIST

A clever version of the 'two-truths-and-a-lie' game

AT A GLANCE
A group attempts to guess which of a set of 'true' statements reflecting the experiences of a small group is, in fact, false.

WHAT YOU NEED
10 – 30 mins (depending on size of groups)

WHAT TO DO
Use a fun random method (see Group-Splitting Exercises on page 32) to divide your gathering into groups of four or five people. It does not matter if the groups are uneven in number, but plenty of room between each group is helpful.

Allow each group five or so minutes to secretly discuss among themselves the things they have in common with one another. Their object is to discover at least three or four 'things' that are common to everyone in their small group, but – and this is the fun bit – one of the 'things' must be false, i.e., this one statement is not common because it does not apply to one or more people in the group.

For example, sharing some statements

I have heard groups make about themselves:

- We have all been to the Melbourne Zoo and had a butterfly land on our heads;
- We have all driven more than 10 kilometres in a car (6 miles) with the hand-brake on;
- None of us have ever broken a bone in our body; and
- We can all sing the first verse of at least three Beatles' songs.

It works best if you encourage lots of creative thoughts to avoid statements like "We all use a toothbrush to clean our teeth" or "We all live in a house." So, provide some good out-of-the-box-thinking examples (like those above) to fire up your group's creative juices.

Then, one at a time, invite each small group to stand, or come before the rest of the group, and with their best dead-pan faces, present their three or four 'truthful' statements. The aim is for everyone else (the jury) to guess which one statement is false. Often, because there is a lot to take in at once, it's OK to ask the small group to make their statements several times.

I have found that developing three or four statements is good, but any more is often too hard.

Got a really large group? Same set-up, just involve more people in each group, and give them a little more time to identify their 'categories.'

Variations

- You could ask each group to simply write their statements on paper, for the rest of the group to read. However, this option will not afford the 'jury' the opportunity to watch their compatriots squirm as they try to keep a straight face and tell a lie.

- As an exercise in decision-making, ask the jury to make a unanimous decision. That is, the group tries to reach consensus on which one of the statements is the lie. As best you try, this technique still often ends up as a vote! That's OK – it's the process that counts – it could provide a useful processing topic for you.

SNOWFLAKE

A simple, creative yet powerful activity that opens people's eyes to being different

AT A GLANCE

With their eyes closed, people follow the instructions of a leader to fold and tear small pieces out of a sheet of paper several times to produce a 'snowflake' shape.

WHAT YOU NEED

Sheet of paper for each person
5 – 10 mins

WHAT TO DO

With a sheet of paper in their hands, ask each person to close their eyes until you ask them to open them. Sometimes, for the benefit of those sneaky folk who just can't resist looking, it's useful to explain that the exercise will take no longer than two minutes.

Before you go any further, clearly explain that you will provide very clear instructions that everyone will hear. However, no one is permitted to ask any questions. None. Encourage your group to solve the problem without speaking. This is very important – you'll see why soon.

You're now ready to make snow. Checking that everyone's eyes are closed (you may keep yours open), clearly give the following instructions, one at a time with appropriate pauses in between:

"FOLD YOUR PAPER IN HALF, AND KEEP IT FOLDED.

TEAR OFF THE BOTTOM RIGHT-HAND CORNER.

DISCARD THE TORN SECTION TO YOUR SIDE.

FOLD YOUR PAPER IN HALF AGAIN, AND KEEP IT FOLDED.

TEAR OFF THE TOP LEFT-HAND CORNER.

DISCARD THE TORN SECTION.

FOLD YOUR PAPER INTO HALF AGAIN, AND KEEP IT FOLDED.

TEAR OFF THE BOTTOM LEFT-HAND CORNER.

DISCARD THE TORN SECTION.

FOLD YOUR PAPER INTO HALF AGAIN, AND KEEP IT FOLDED.

USING YOUR TEETH, TEAR OFF THE TOP RIGHT-HAND CORNER.

FOR THE FINAL TIME, FOLD YOUR PAPER IN HALF DIAGONALLY AND PRESS ON THE FOLD AS BEST YOU CAN.

YOU MAY NOW OPEN YOUR EYES."

Note: I recommend completing at least four folds, preferably five, to give the best results. Though, I will admit that the fourth and final tear is a doozy. That's why the teeth come in handy.

Now, sit back and take in the range of reactions you will have generated. "Yours is different to mine," "I've screwed it up," "Mine looks so pretty," "Hey?," etc, the whole gamut. As a fun little exercise you could leave it here, but I would strongly recommend taking a few minutes to process the outcome.

You could ask questions such as:

- Why does everyone's creation look different?

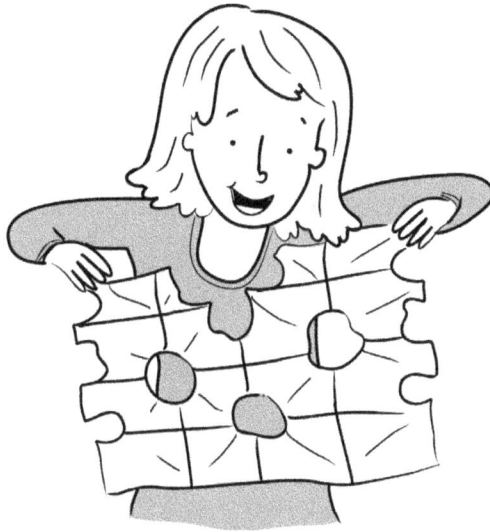

- What was the first question you wanted to ask, if you could have? What was the second, etc?
- Whose design is the right one?
- What might this result suggest in terms of how this group may work together?
- What are the strengths and limitations of everyone being different?
- What impact does this knowledge have on your performance as a group?

Clearly, the analogy is that like a snowflake, we are all different. We hear things differently; we all see things from diverse perspectives, etc, etc. Also, from the perspective of teamwork, a snowball (all the flakes working together) is much more powerful than a single snowflake. Tie these threads into your conversation, and you will likely see a few pennies drop.

Variation

Involve the use of scissors and create extraordinarily intricate snowflake designs. Just ask people to be careful as they do the cutting.

TALKING BEHIND YOUR BACK

A get-to-know-you-better activity that is affirming as much as it is energising

AT A GLANCE

Individuals mingle about an area with an index card taped to their back, inviting others to write positive comments on the card.

WHAT YOU NEED

Large index card, and a pen for each person
Sticky-tape
5 – 10 mins

WHAT TO DO

Here's a great energiser that is not only quick and fun, but great for groups who already know a lot about each other.

Distribute a large index card and a pen to each person, and ask them to write their name on the top of the card. Using a slip of sticky-tape, and possibly the help of a friend, fix the card to its owner's back. You could use a sheet of paper, but I have often found that it's not quite thick enough to prevent the occasional pen from penetrating the paper, and therefore the clothing behind it.

Ask your group to mingle about the area armed with pens. Their mission is to approach as many people as possible in the time allotted and write a short remark or comment on their cards. It should go without saying, but you often have to – the remarks should aim to be life-affirming and positive. Funny is okay, so long as the recipient would laugh along too.

Time's up. Remove all of the cards, and either invite each person to read the comments, or better still – lay all of the cards out on the floor or a table, and allow the group to browse them. People will quickly appreciate how others feel about them, a wonderfully affirming experience.

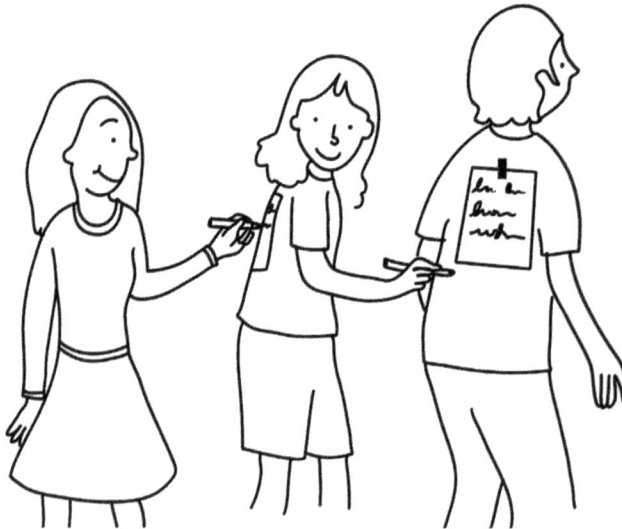

Variations

- Before the cards are removed, ask each person to ruminate out loud what they think may have been written on their cards. This is an awesome challenge for some folks, so a personal favourite.

- Original format, but this time, stick the index card on backwards so the name does not show. Then before their owners get to see them, someone (often the leader) removes all of the cards, shuffles them, and lays them out for everyone to view (owner's names face-down). The object is for each person to guess which card is theirs.

ACE OF SPADES

A brilliant 'luck-of-the-draw' mixer

AT A GLANCE

On an agreed signal, people quickly pair up and form one of three physical poses with another person in their group, hoping it is not the pose randomly chosen by the leader to eliminate people.

WHAT YOU NEED

Deck of playing cards, including Jokers
5 – 10 mins

WHAT TO DO

See Snappy Partners (page 34) for a great group-splitting activity that leads brilliantly into this one.

Pull the four Aces and one of the two Jokers from a regular playing deck of cards. Shuffle the cards (you'll come back to them later), and then ask your group to mingle about a defined area. No talking, no touching, just wandering aimlessly around.

Then upon an agreed signal, such as "STOP" or when the music is paused (if you are so disposed), explain that everyone must find a partner as quickly as possible and form one of three phys-

ical gestures or poses. The pose can be whatever you like – maybe even relate them to your group in some meaningful way – it doesn't matter, as long as everyone is clear about what their options are.

I have often chosen the following poses:

- Partners stand back to back
- Partners embrace in a mutual hug
- One person sits on the knee of their kneeling partner.

Other options include: linking elbows, holding hands, or for the more physically inclined, having one person piggyback the other, or for one person to carry the other in his or her arms.

This is what happens. People mingle, mingle, mingle, until the call to "STOP" is given, and there is suddenly a rush as people chase down partners. They quickly concur to form one of the three poses, and then a card is pulled randomly from your hand of shuffled cards as they await the result. You see, each card represents a particular pose, such as:

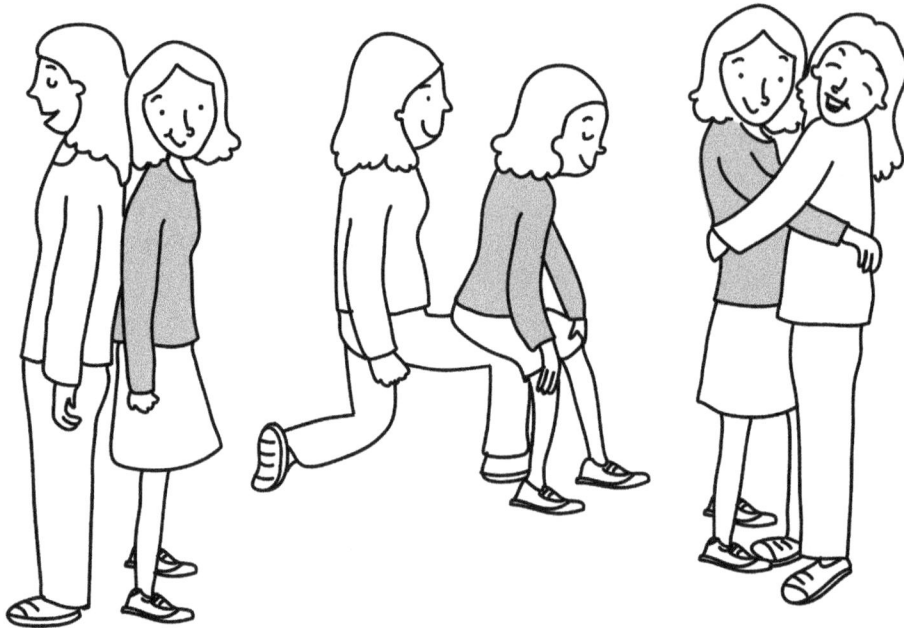

Ace of Clubs – one person sits on partner's knee

Ace of Diamonds – partners stand back to back

Ace of Hearts – partners hug

So, when a particular card is drawn, everyone matching that pose is asked to sign off and enjoy the continuing action from the sidelines. However, if the Ace of Spades is drawn, nothing happens, and everyone resumes their mingling happy in the knowledge that they lasted one more round. If the Joker is pulled, everyone is back in the game. Woo hoo! Game continues until you are left with one very lucky pair.

Encourage people to look for a new partner each time they form a pose. If you wish, every now and then invite the various couples to share something about themselves.

Variations

- As above, but invite people to stick with the same partner for each round. They simply re-locate each other at the conclusion of each round of mingling.

- Rather than eliminate those pairs that match the drawn card, these folks survive to live another round. A 'winner' will emerge much more quickly this way.

THUMB WRESTLING IN STEREO

Fantastic variation on an old favourite

AT A GLANCE
Partners form a 'monkey-grip' with their hands, and each tries to pin the other person's thumb under their own first.

WHAT YOU NEED
5 - 10 mins

WHAT TO DO
Ask your group to separate into pairs. Using the same hand, instruct each person to hold their partner's hand as if in the typical 'monkey-grip' position, i.e., fingers curled into the palm of the other. At this juncture, you could simply launch into wrestle mania, but try these two fun adaptations to add a little pizzazz to an otherwise I-can-see-what's-going-to-happen activity:

- Ask each person to grasp the free hand of their partner to form a second 'combat zone' situated on top of or below their already coupled hands. Their arms should now looked crossed, to give that peculiar stereo look.

- Suggest that before play commences, the partners should join in a quick preparative ditty of "One, two, three, four; I declare a thumb war," during which the opposing thumbs alternate side to side across their respective corners of the 'playing field.'

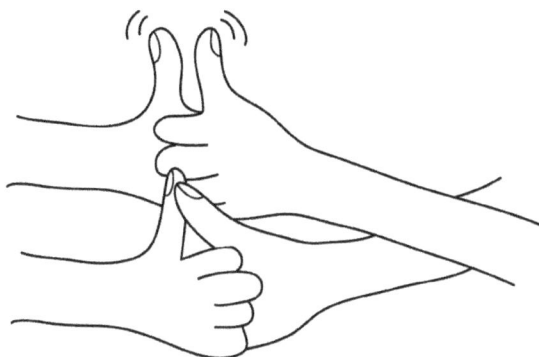

You are now primed to engage in mortal thumb combat. The object is to pin your partner's thumb under your own first. Note: Slipping out from under your partner's thumb, after having been momentarily pinned, is a breach of the International Thumb Wrestling Convention! Let the games begin.

Variations

- Swap the set of hands that appears on top of the other.
- Try it with three or four people. Continue to apply the 'monkey-grip' posture, but this time all wrestlers curl their fingers in one big clump of palm propinquity. Opportunities to form alliances (i.e., "Let's work together to pin HIS thumb first.") adds another level of excitement to the game.

ESP

A mind-reading exercise that's full of fun and surprises

AT A GLANCE

Starting back to back, pairs turn around to face their partners and physically demonstrate one of three gestures, aiming to match their partner's gesture.

WHAT YOU NEED

10 - 15 mins

WHAT TO DO

Separate your group into pairs and then conduct a whole group discussion that will result in an agreement of three definable, distinct physical gestures. Your program goals will dictate what style of gestures they will be; for example, a recreational program may settle with three popular sporting movements such as a golf swing, swimming and horse-riding (to save space, you'll just have to imagine what these movements look like).

Alternatively, for programs of a more intrinsic nature, you could come up with happy, sad and shocked featuring commonly accepted gestures for each of them. It doesn't matter too much, but I encourage you to motivate the group to develop the gestures, with you as the final arbiter of what is appropriate, of course!

Practice these gestures a few times to ensure that everyone has got them locked in. Now ask each of the pairs to find a little space to play, and stand back to back with their partners, i.e., so that they can't see each other. Whilst waiting for the countdown, each person is silently deciding which of the three gestures he or she will choose to do. No talking or giving of clues is permitted during this period.

Then, on the count of three, each person turns around swiftly to face their partner whilst demonstrating / performing one of the three gestures. A clue – instruct people to be gesturing as they turn around, to prevent a little sneaky cheating. The object of each pair is to match gestures, e.g., a swimmer faces another swimmer. Strangely, wild screams of delight emanate from the pairs regardless of whether they match or not.

Repeat this procedure five or six times, suggesting that each partnership tally their results. Upon the final round, survey your group for the most perceptive couples! It's not rare to find that some partnerships earn a perfect record, but it is certainly not common. What does this mean? Hmmm, I'll leave that to your debrief, but a high degree of success among many of the pairs may reflect a high level of connectedness within the group. Or just plain luck!

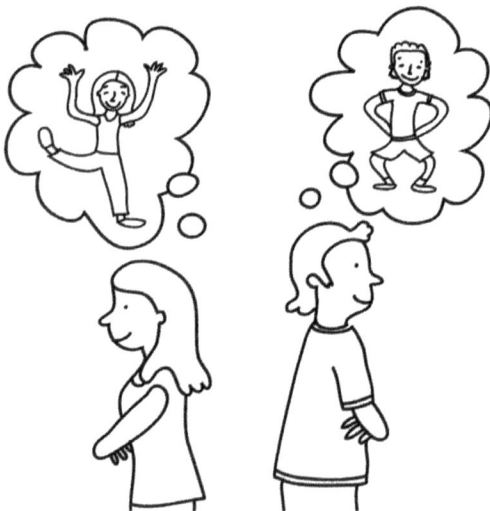

Variations

- Use groups of three people; tougher to match, but same deal.
- Introduce four or perhaps even five distinct gestures.
- Use as a fun way to introduce an important component of your program; for example, the Full Value Contract where you facilitate the group to create a distinct physical gesture for each element of the agreement.

SPOT THE DIFFERENCE

A classic observation exercise that's all about subtleties

AT A GLANCE

Upon turning to face their partners, having had their back to them for a minute, each person attempts to spot as many changes in the appearance of their partner as possible.

WHAT YOU NEED
10 – 20 mins

WHAT TO DO

Ideal for slowing the pace of your program, and to encourage your group to notice the subtle things about other people that we often overlook.

You need pairs. Try a group-splitting exercise from pages 32 to 41. Ask each pair to start by standing back to back with their partner. It's important that you do not telegraph what you are about to do in advance of this step, for reasons that will soon become obvious.

Next, instruct each person to change or alter three things about their appearance during the next 60 seconds – without sneaking a peek! No need to give them examples of what to change – they always work it out. Swap a watch to the other wrist, fold up cuffs, unbutton a shirt. The key is that all changes have to be visible, so moving the lint from one pocket to another doesn't fly.

Time's up. Now ask each person to spin around, face their partner, and taking turns, identify all of the changes that have been made.

Now for stage two. Return the pairs to their original back-to-back stances, and ask them to change three more things about their appearance. Once you get past the initial groans of "What, another three?," your group will soon discover that there are an endless number of changes they can make by adding to themselves, and not just taking away.

You could probably squeeze another three changes if you wanted, at which point, some people are reduced to subtle and not-so-subtle changes in their facial appearance! A classic.

Variation

Establish groups of four (or six), where two (or three) people work to identify the changes in another two (or three) people.

BOUNCEY BOUNCEY

Utterly crazy, yet a quick and easy partner energiser

AT A GLANCE
Standing back to back, two people connect with one another and bounce up and down a pre-determined number of times.

WHAT YOU NEED
1 minute

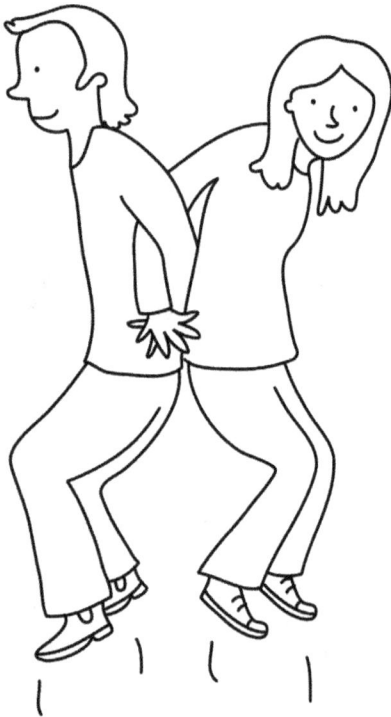

WHAT TO DO
This has got to be one of the craziest games I think I have ever come across, but it works like a charm.

Separate into pairs, perhaps locating a partner who is of similar height. Ask each person to choose a number between 1 and 5, share it with their partner, and then calculate the sum.

Next, ask the pairs to turn back to back, and interlock their elbows with one another to form a cosy connection. Finally, announce that you would like each partnership to bounce up and down together according to the sum they generated. One (up), two (up), three (up) …

Crazy, I know. But I guarantee, it will energise your group, not to mention create lots of laughter.

If you sense that some participants may find it difficult to lock elbows (or may not be careful in their pursuit of bounces), suggest that they may choose to hold hands while standing back-to-back.

Hint: do not telegraph what you are about to ask the pairs to do. Preserve the adventure for as long as possible. If you happen to describe what you are about to ask the pairs to do before you ask them to choose a number, most savvy folks will cotton on and aim low.

Variations

- Each person picks a number from 1 to 10.

- Form groups of three, four or whatever number of people. With groups of four or more, you can invite people to turn to face each other (or not), then jump.

OFF BALANCE

A great physical exercise to build harmony, trust and support

AT A GLANCE
Two people invent and attempt as many unusual ways to physically balance off one another, while also supporting each other.

WHAT YOU NEED
2 – 5 mins

WHAT TO DO
Like Moon Walking and Human Spring in the pages prior, you need to present this wonderfully inventive activity in the correct sequence. Out of place, and you risk hurting people. But let's not go overboard with the warnings – this exercise is not all that dangerous and can be done quite safely. Remember, your approach is everything.

Everyone finds a partner who, let's say, is as tall as they are. To begin, ask each person to stand facing their partner and firmly grasp their hands or wrists, whatever is most comfortable. Next, announce that you want them to invent as many crazy, off-balance positions as they can think of in which each person is leaning backwards to the point that if it weren't for his or her partner, they would fall in a heap on the ground.

Make a few comments about not placing too much strain or pressure on their partners, and keeping a safe distance from other couples and certain eye-gouging protrusions. Then – this is the hard part – stand back, and leave the rest up to your group's imagination.

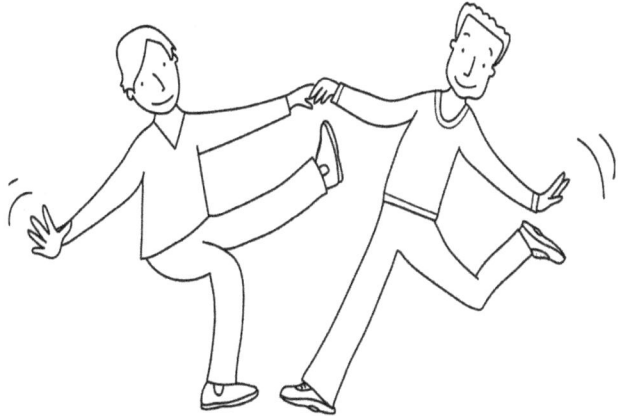

Framed correctly, you will observe some extraordinarily, harmonious working relationships develop. Mingle among the balance-impaired and encourage them to explore different balance points of the body – one leg, back-to-back, tippy-toes, etc. There's no right answer – it's all about learning to play, support and trust.

Variation

Invite one couple to join with another to form a group of four people, performing similar off-balanced feats of engineering.

FINGER FENCING

Try this out for some swash-buckling fun and interaction.

AT A GLANCE

Two people, connected by their right hands with their index fingers extended, attempt to be the first to tag the other below the waist.

WHAT YOU NEED

5 mins

WHAT TO DO

Ask everyone to find a suitable 'Errol Flynn' partner and a space to engage in a grand duel. Invite one promising 'swash-buckler' to step forward to help you demonstrate this exercise.

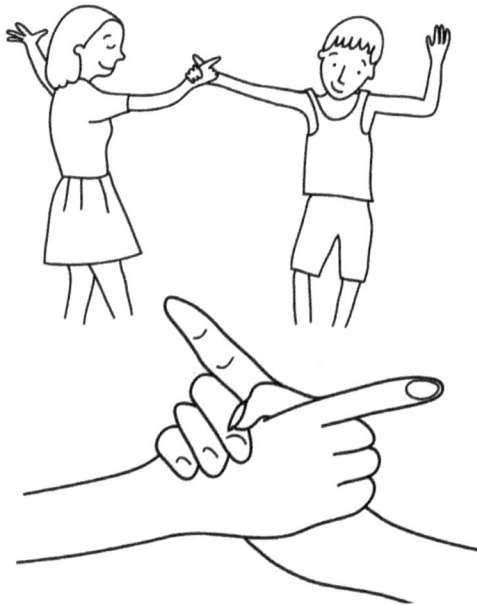

This is where your zany over-the-top impression of Errol Flynn will impress everyone to give it a go. First, you need to dress for the part, so slip into your fencing suit, put on your mask, and 'swish-swish' your foil. Bow to your partner, and then extend both of your right hands forward to join in one of those funky handshakes, you know, those cool clasp-your-partner's-thumb-on-top handshakes. From this position, you each extend your index finger out as if you were pointing down the forearm of your partner. Announce with a flourish that this finger is... your foil.

Place your other hand elegantly in the air behind you a la sixteenth-century style, turn side-on and lift the toe of your front foot, and voila – you're ready to engage in 'mortal combat.'

With a call of "ON GUARD!" the match begins. Feet shuffle and foils swish everywhere. The first person to touch the other with their finger (foil) somewhere on the body below their waist (and beyond their wrist), exclaims "TOUCHÉ" and is declared the winner.

Variations

- Use your left arm to create the foil.
- Designate a tight boundary inside which the action can take place. If someone steps outside the boundary, they are considered tagged.
- Double the trouble! While attempting to tag your opponent with your finger, try to tag one of their feet with your foot as well.

TOE TAG

A hop-step-and-jump tag game that quickly raises the energy of your group

AT A GLANCE

Starting back to back, two partners spin around on "GO" and try to tag the toe of their partner before they get tagged.

WHAT YOU NEED

2 – 5 mins

WHAT TO DO

This is a perfect two-minute filler that has the power to transform your mopey group into a ball of energy. You need groups made up of partners. Ask everyone to start with their backs to their partners, and on an appropriate signal like "GO," both partners spin around 180 degrees to face one another and engage in a dance-like combat.

Each person attempts to 'tag' the toe of their partner gently before one of their own feet gets tagged. Be sure to remind your group that you said "tagged" and not "stomped." This will make all the difference between many fun rounds, and a lot of sore feet. Play best of three rounds, but if you lose the first two, better make it five!

Variations

- If too much energy is expended chasing your partner, a less aerobic version is to start by facing your partner and holding his or her hands.

- Form a circle with your group holding hands. Each person attempts to tag the feet of their immediate neighbours. As soon as a person has had both feet tagged, they retreat from the circle. The group re-joins, and the game continues until the final two 'toe-taggers' duel.

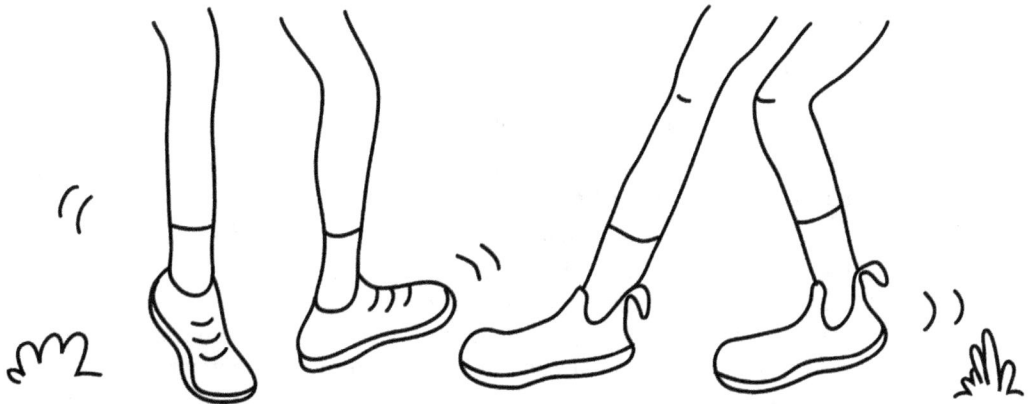

SQUAT THRUST

One of those simple, but oh-so-hard-to-balance exercises

AT A GLANCE

Two people, facing one another about 60 cm (2') apart, squat down on the balls of their feet, and attempt to bring their partner off balance using only their hands as a point of contact.

WHAT YOU NEED

A 2 - 3 metre (10') rope for each pair (optional)

2 – 5 mins

WHAT TO DO

Announce that you would like everyone to find a partner who has similarly-sized hands. After genial greetings are exchanged, you ask each person to face their partner and to stand about 60 cm (2') apart – as measured from toe to toe. With feet together, demonstrate the required pose by squatting down, bending at the knees, teetering on the balls of your feet. With hands in the 'bumpers-up' position, i.e., hands up, palms facing forward in front of you, you are now ready to engage.

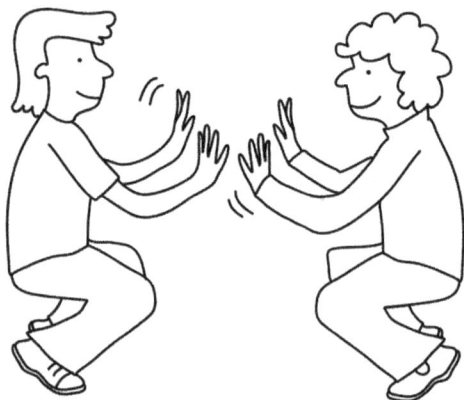

On "GO" – because it's a great way to start a game – explain that the goal is for each person to bring their partner off balance (notice, I did not say "Push your buddy over"). Oh, and to make it a little more interesting, explain that the only area of the body that can be touched is the hands. That's right, a person is not entitled to touch any other anatomical part of their opponent to cause them to come off balance. Oftentimes, a touch is not even necessary to cause a toppling over; a good baulk is always clever.

Make it best out of three, and at some suitable point, invite everyone to find a new sparring partner and start over.

Variations

- Restrict each person to the use of one hand only.

- Divide into groups of four people, squatting in a square-like formation. Now it's every person for him or her self.

- Original set-up, but this time the partners hold a short rope, approx 2 - 3 metres (7 – 10') between them. Squatting about a metre apart (3'), their object is to use the rope (push, pull or otherwise) to cause their partner to come off balance. To keep it safe, encourage people to hold their end of the rope inside their palm only, and not to wrap it around their wrists.

MOON WALKING

The closest people can get to flying without wings

AT A GLANCE

Two people holding the lower arms of a third person whose hands are on his or her hips, physically support the latter as he or she jumps into the air.

WHAT YOU NEED

2 – 5 mins

WHAT TO DO

Use a variety of Clumps (see page 33), ending with "THREE" to form random groups of three people. Ask one person to place hands on hips (thumbs pointing backwards) and to hold this stance firm. Instruct the two others of this triad to approach the first person, and grab a lower arm each with their two hands, often placing one hand at the wrist and the other just below the elbow.

Upon engaging in this exercise, allow people to choose where is best for them to place their hands. What is important to stress, however, is gentle but firm grips, and that the middle person maintains a solid stance at all times.

Now, commence the countdown, and ask each of the middle people to jump high into the air. At the same time, their partners will lift their colleagues

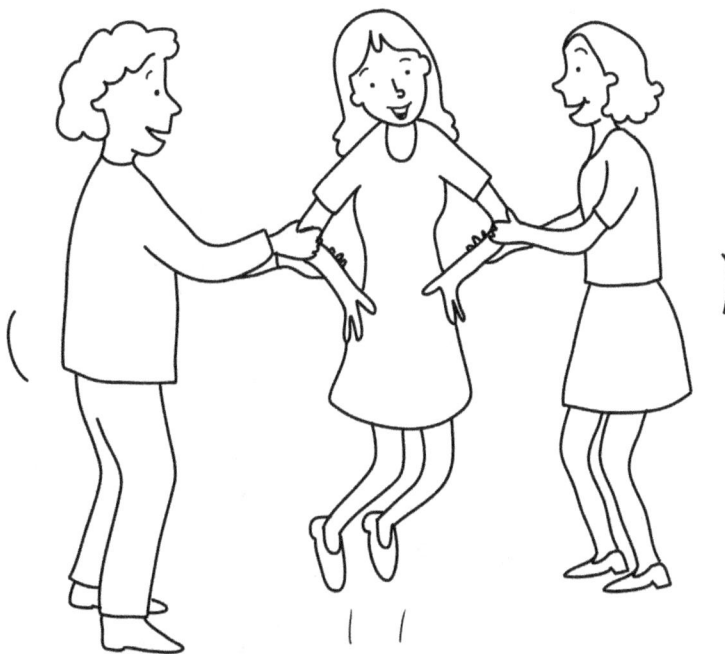

gently into the air giving extra support to allow for a jump which is higher than can normally be expected. Note, I said "gently" and "extra support" – not fling, heave or toss your jumper into the air!

Depending on your sequence, this could be one of the first occasions in which you have introduced some form of exhilarating physical rush for your participants. It will often elicit much applause and screams (of joy). Apart from the obvious merriment of jumping really high, this is also an excellent activity to introduce your group to the concept of taking care of others – which, in turn, contributes to building a feeling of trust, support and community.

Hence, your sequencing must be spot on. Do not introduce this exercise to your group unless they have already exhibited healthy levels of safety consciousness in your lead-up activities.

Variation

Same set-up as above, but this time, invite the threesome to move forward five paces, stepping forward in rapid succession with each jump. It will almost feel like flying.

HUMAN SPRING

An exciting, physical exercise that will test your group's adroitness

AT A GLANCE

Two people facing each other, with open palms stretched slightly forward, lean into one another simultaneously and break their respective falls as their hands meet in the middle.

WHAT YOU NEED

2 – 5 mins

WHAT TO DO

As a rather physically-involved activity, sequence this one appropriately. Some warm-ups, stretches or the like would be ideal, but consider the emotional readiness of your group as well.

Separate your group into pairs, and invite each partnership to face one another standing about 60 cm (2 feet) apart. Ask them to raise their hands, with their open palms facing toward their partner. Now explain that you would like each person to slowly – let me say that again, slowly – lean in toward their partner until their hands meet in the middle. With arms bent, the meeting of hands will feel quite springy, and it's supposed to. But if heads smash, there's too much give in the springs!

From this position, invite each partnership to spring off one another by pushing away from the other. With a little practice, and timed perfectly, a couple can lean in, spring back, lean in and spring back effortlessly for a long time. That's the goal, to develop a rhythm and tune into the partner's body and needs. To push a mate over is not. Accordingly, keep a watchful eye on proceedings, and if you catch a few too many over-zealous attempts, step in and adjust.

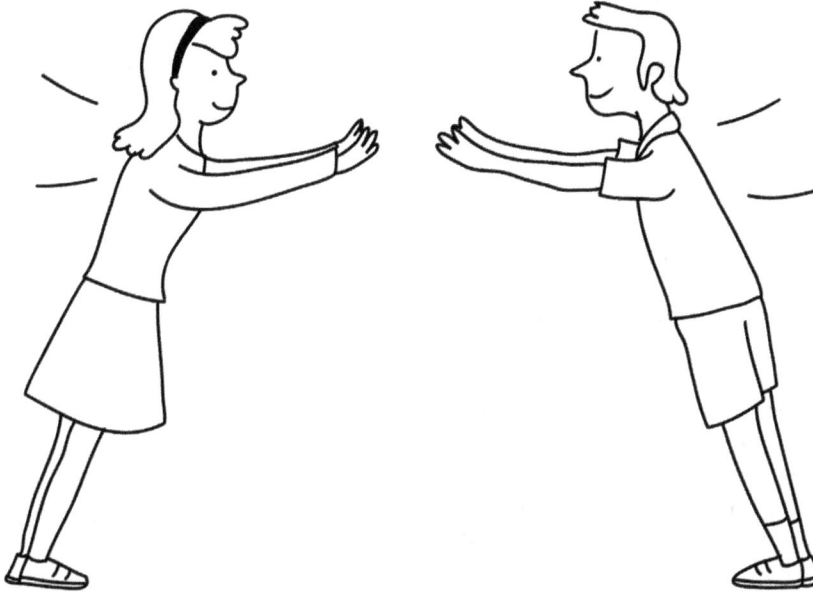

Variations

- Picking your moment, invite each springing duo to try one or more of the following variations:
  - Take a step further away from each other.
  - Use only one hand.
  - Use both hands, but cross your two arms.
  - Cross your legs.

CLAPPING GAME

A sure-fire energiser that will raise the energy of your group, and make 'em laugh

AT A GLANCE

Standing in front of a group, one person passes their hands in front of themselves in a repeated back and forth motion asking everyone to clap only when his or her hands pass.

WHAT YOU NEED

1 – 2 mins

WHAT TO DO

You need one person to stand in front of your group. Maybe that's you? Explain that you want everyone to watch carefully as you move your hands back and forth in a particular pattern. Perhaps alternating left and right, or up and down, it doesn't matter much. Just make sure that at some point your hands cross during the journey.

The fun part is that you ask your group to clap every time they see your hands cross. It's at this point, I rediscover how much I love this game, energiser, diversion, call it what you like. The intense focus and concentration on people's faces is priceless.

So you start passing, slow at first, then in rapid succession. And then, I suggest, you get tricky. Make out like your hands are about to cross, but they don't. Guaranteed, money in the bank, this lark will cause your group to clap, and then quickly realising their mistake, laugh out loud.

You need only present this exercise for minute or so, and it will produce the desired effect. Your group will now be bubbling with more energy, and there will be smiles and laughter aplenty.

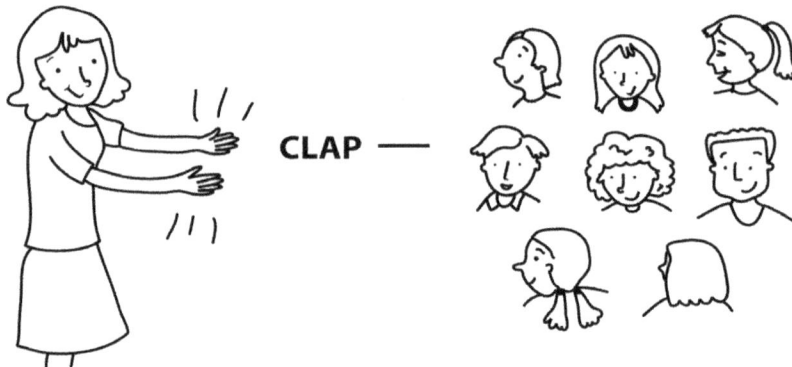

CLAP —

Variation

Structured as an elimination game, same rules apply. If someone makes a 'mistake,' for example, a person claps when they shouldn't, or is late, etc, they are asked to step aside, sit down or whatever and enjoy the continuing action. Keep going until one person remains, and give them a round of applause!

GOTCHA

Never fails to produce raptures of laughter

AT A GLANCE

Standing in a circle with their index fingers pointing downward into their partners' open palms, everyone tries to catch the juxtapositioned finger at the same time.

WHAT YOU NEED

5 - 10 mins

WHAT TO DO

Ask your group to form a circle, facing inwards and standing side by side. (Note, this next bit is best if you demonstrate as you explain it.) Holding your right hand out to your right hand side (about shoulder height) with your palm facing upwards, extend the index finger of your left hand, and place it into the open palm of the person on your left.

Look around, and you should all be inextricably linked. Now, on the command "GO!" – which works pretty well to start a game – everyone tries to catch the finger of the person on their right, that which is pointing downward, touching the centre of their palm. Of course, jocularity prevails, because everyone is also trying to avoid being caught by the person on their left. I just love that bit. Ask people to shout out "GOTCHA!" when they catch a finger.

Now, you could try to move on, but I doubt you will want to. There are ample moments of humour here. Observe the way in which the palms of some people that started out as flat are slowly curling with each round. Or the proclivity of folks to not want to touch their finger tip on their neighbour's palm, lest they get caught!! It's all so funny.

My biggest Gotcha group? Two-hundred and fifty! Spectacular.

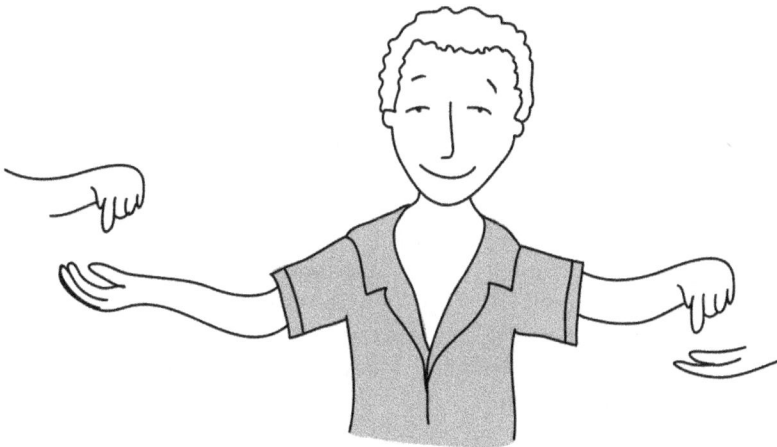

Variations

- Try this again several times, switching palms from the right to the left (to benefit our left-brained friends), i.e., the left palm is facing upwards, and a right index finger is extended.

- Cross your arms as you play, i.e., extend the right palm in front of your chest to point toward the person on your left, and place your left index finger into the waiting palm on your right.

- Try all variations with your palms upside-down, and index fingers pointing up.

- Regular set-up, but this time each person attempts to catch the finger sitting in their right palm with their left hand. Try it. Hilarious.

- Original set-up, add a further challenge. Instruct people to place their right foot directly above, but not touching the left toes of their right-hand side partner. On "GO," you try to tag the foot of your partner, whilst trying to avoid being tagged and performing the usual finger and palm routine.

- Everything above, but groups of only two or three or whatever.

GALLOPING HANDS

A quick one-minute energiser that's sure to get hearts beating

AT A GLANCE
Sitting in a circle, individuals slap their open hands on their laps as quickly as possible after their neighbours have just slapped their hands.

WHAT YOU NEED
Two soft objects (optional)
1 – 2 mins

WHAT TO DO
Got a group sitting in a circle, wondering what to do to fill in some time, or perhaps needing a little pep?

Ask everyone to place their open hands (palms facing down) onto their lap. Then, having agreed on a suitable starting routine ("1, 2, 3" or "READY-SET-GO," etc), you explain that you want a sequence of hands being slapped on laps around the circle (direction is up to you) occurring at break-neck speed. Not really fast, not even dynamically speedy – but break-neck speed. Ham it up ... you get the idea.

Then with your typical flourish, begin the sequence by slapping your own lap, and henceforth set off an impulse of slaps around the circle. Time it if you will, but everyone will know without a stop-watch if you have (or have not) achieved the desired velocity. Repeat several times. Go both directions to check which route is fastest.

Why break-neck speed? Observe people's heads as they watch the impulse pass them by. Enough said.

Variations

- Invite people to place one hand each on the knee of their two closest neighbours, i.e., your left hand rests on the right knee of your left-hand neighbour, and vice versa. This time the impulse is created by consecutive hands as governed by the sequence of knees.

- Send an impulse of claps around the circle, break neck speed of course!

BEAT THE BUNNY

Simple energiser that's an ideal follow-on from Galloping Hands

AT A GLANCE
Sitting in a circle, individuals pass one small object as quickly as possible to their neighbour in an attempt to 'catch' a second object also being passed in the same direction.

WHAT YOU NEED
Two soft objects (optional)
1 – 2 mins

WHAT TO DO
Most often, your group will be seated, however, it works just as well standing up.

Introduce two small soft objects, such as two different coloured balls or two beanie babies. Pass one item around the circle from person to person as quickly as possible, and stop it when it reaches the half way point. Compliment the group for their speed, but suggest that they can still move the object much more quickly. Think 'break neck' speed (see Galloping Hands page 88).

Now, introduce the second object. Explain that this object is Farmer Brown, and the first half-way positioned object is the bunny. Farmer Brown doesn't like

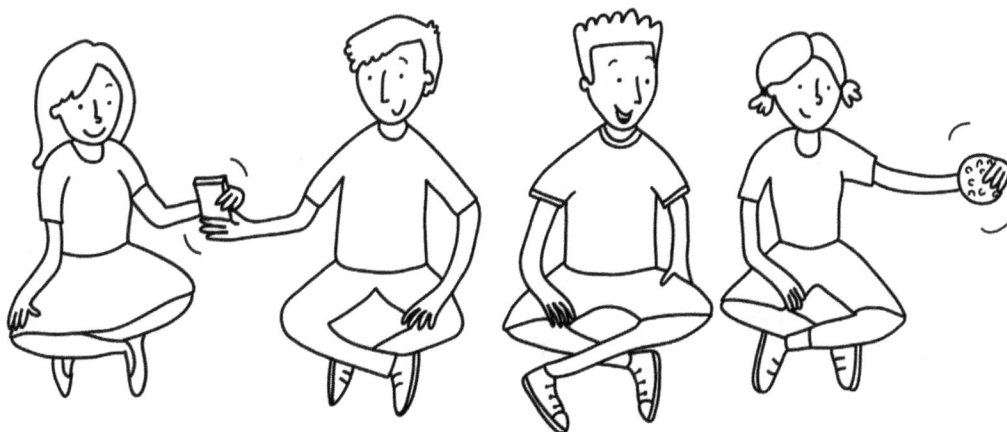

bunnies, so he's going to chase it. And off you go, passing the second object in the same direction as the bunny is travelling. The goal is for the farmer to chase the bunny down and touch it. Sounds simple? It's not.

To make it a little more interesting, allow Farmer Brown to change his direction at any time. The bunny can never choose to change direction, unless and until the farmer has changed his direction.

Variation

For really large groups, introduce many objects (call them what you like), have them all travel in the same direction. The goal is for any object to draw near to and touch any object ahead of it.

FILL THE SPACE

Perfect for large groups, promoting lots of fun and non-threatening interaction

AT A GLANCE

People mingle in a space, responding to instructions to follow, lead and evade certain other people.

WHAT YOU NEED

5 – 10 mins

WHAT TO DO

Invite your group to spread out randomly but evenly inside an area that you have designated. Ask each person to slowly mingle about the area and attempt to "fill the (empty) spaces" as they are created here and there. Suggest that there is no need for talking or touching. Ask that participants simply move and observe all that is around them. Indeed, with a very large group, it is important that they refrain from chitter-chatter.

As your group has started to mill about (notice, how funny your group will think this is already!), call out to ask each person to secretly identify someone on the other side of the space. That other person doesn't know that they have been chosen. Then ask participants to follow as closely behind that secret person as is possible – so that each time he or she moves away, they must follow.

Obviously (and you don't need to say this), this is a set-up, because everyone is following a different person. They frantically move about to catch up with their ever-moving targets. Maintaining a walking pace is important though – there are always one or two who insist on mingling 'briskly,' otherwise known as running.

After a few moments, ask the group to resume their mingling, and repeat the process with a new secret admirer. Or, move on to one of the following variations.

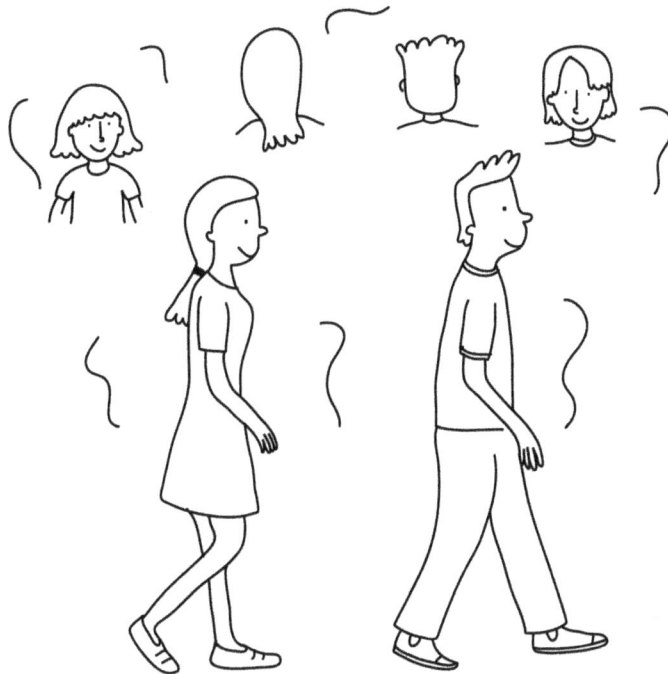

Variations

- Say to participants:
  - "As you mingle, secretly identify a person close to you, and then keep as far away as possible (within the boundaries) from this person.
  - Select a person on the other side again, and then try to keep an equal distance in front of them at all times. As a further twist, make sure this other person notices you!
  - Secretly identify two people, one of whom you will attempt to keep between you and the other secret person at all times – as if you were hiding behind the former so as not to be seen by the latter. Painfully difficult, but extraordinarily fun."

STOP & GO

Great exercise to give your participants a chance to control the flow of a game

AT A GLANCE

People walk about a defined area and respond immediately when anyone from the group calls out "STOP" and "GO."

WHAT YOU NEED

3 to 5 mins

WHAT TO DO

This is way simple. First, designate a general area where your group is permitted to walk about aimlessly. I say "general" because who cares if someone decides to step outside the boundaries? There's no penalty, and it has no impact on the game. Therefore, there is little need for boundary markers and the like, but feel free to use them; it makes no matter. What does matter, is that people walk, not run.

Explain that as everyone is milling about, anyone may at any time shout out either "STOP" to force everyone to freeze immediately where they are, or "GO" to have them resume their walking. That's it. Do this for a few minutes. It's a great warm-up, and builds energy quickly.

I love watching my group as they trade their respective "STOP"s and "GO"s. You can learn a lot in these few minutes. It's up to the interaction of the group to make the game work.

So, having given up the leadership, how do you end the game? Many choices, but two of my favourites are to either just step in and say, "OK, that's enough;" or suggest that whenever five or more people remain frozen after the

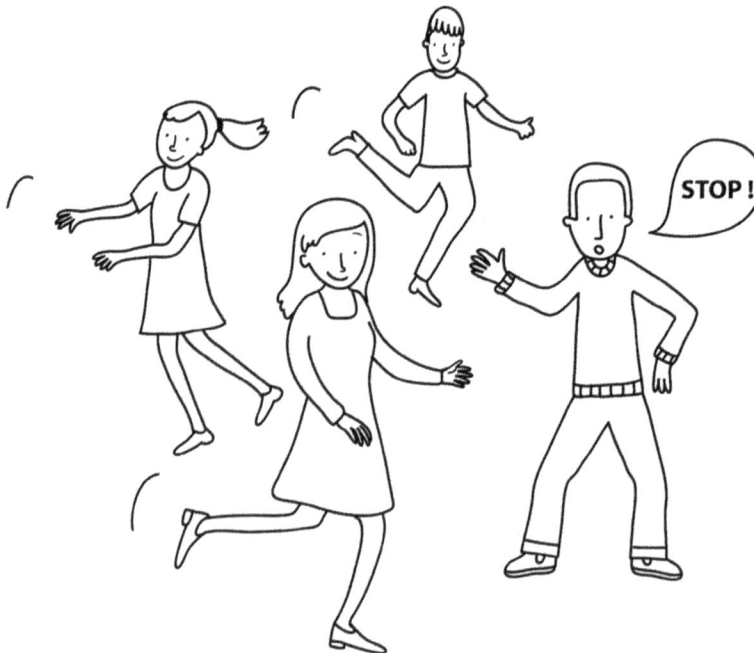

call for "GO," the game is over.

Something to look for – often, after the group has been milling about for some time, two or more people will shout out instantaneously as if triggered by a peculiar chemistry! Always generates lots of laughter.

Variations

- Introduce a variety of calls to mix it up. Try "SLOW MOTION," "BACKWARDS," "HANDS IN THE AIR," "BABY STEPS," and "CLOCKWISE." Invite your group to come up with their own ideas as well.

- To encourage everyone's participation, explain that each person is entitled to make one call only. After a few minutes, most people will have contributed.

MR & MRS WRIGHT

A classic 'listen-to-the-story' energiser

AT A GLANCE

Standing in front of a story-teller, a group will collectively step to the left or right every time they hear the words "LEFT" and "RIGHT" spoken in the story.

WHAT YOU NEED

2 – 4 mins

WHAT TO DO

A simple set-up. Ask your group to stand, finding a space with a little room about them, and to listen closely to a story you are about to narrate. If it's your first time, it's OK to read the story off this page, but as you gain more confidence, you'll be able to make one up on the spot.

The key is, every time you say the word "LEFT," everyone will take a step to the left, and when you say "RIGHT," they step to the right. There are tons of variations of the 'story.' Here's the one I grew up with...

"I'd like to tell you a story about Mr & Mrs WRIGHT.

One evening they were baking cookies and Mrs WRIGHT suddenly called out, "Oh, no, there is no flour LEFT! You will need to go out to the store RIGHT now."

"I can't believe you forgot to check the pantry," grumbled MR WRIGHT.

"It will only take twenty minutes if you come RIGHT back. Go to the corner of First & Second Streets, and turn LEFT at the stop sign. Then go to Forty-Third Street and turn RIGHT, and the shop will be on your LEFT," declared Mrs WRIGHT as her husband LEFT the house.

Mr WRIGHT found the store and asked the assistant where he could find the flour.

The assistant pointed and said, "Go to aisle four and turn LEFT. The flour and sugar will be on your LEFT."

Mr WRIGHT made his purchase and walked RIGHT out the door.

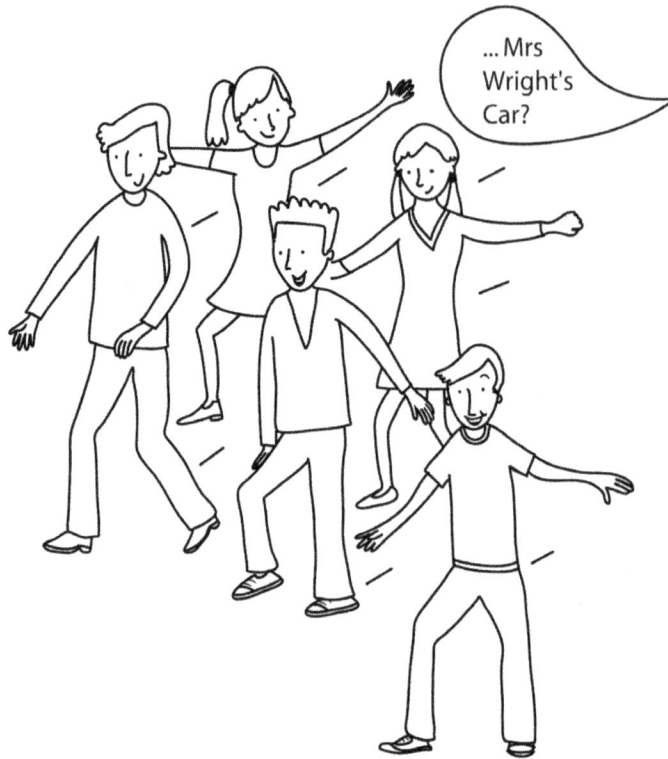

...Mrs Wright's Car?

He turned LEFT, but he couldn't remember where he had LEFT his car.

Suddenly he remembered that he had driven Mrs WRIGHT'S car and that his car was in the driveway at home RIGHT where he had LEFT it.

He finally found the RIGHT car, opened the boot and put the flour RIGHT inside.

Eventually, a weary Mr WRIGHT found his way home.

Mrs WRIGHT had been waiting impatiently. "I thought you would be RIGHT back," she said. "I LEFT all the cookie ingredients on the kitchen counter, and the cats got into the milk. You'll just have to go RIGHT back to the shop again."

Mr WRIGHT sighed. He had no energy LEFT. "I am going RIGHT to bed," he said, and LEFT Mrs WRIGHT standing in the kitchen..."

Variations

- Tell the story with your group standing in a circle. People often mis-step, so the consequences of being in a circle are immediate and hilarious.

- Tell a story that also involves the words UP and DOWN, where people move one step forward or one step back.

RO-SHAM-BO CONGO

Ramping up the fun of an oldie but a goodie

AT A GLANCE

Upon engaging in a quick hand-game duel, winning partners invite their opponents to follow behind them 'congo' style as they continue to play on, aiming to build the longest congo-line possible.

WHAT YOU NEED

2 – 5 mins

WHAT TO DO

Old becomes new with just one simple addition.

First, establish your 'rock-paper-scissors' protocol, because over the years I have found that not everyone plays the same way as I do. Me? I like the standard thrashing of clenched fists into the open palm of my other hand as I call "ONE, TWO, THREE" and on "THREE" I shoot with either a rock (fist remains clenched), paper (hand out flat) or scissors (side-angled peace sign). It doesn't matter what you go with in terms of the count, just as long as everyone knows what's cool today.

Although I accept that the arguments for the orthodox results are kinda flimsy, for those among us who are not 'down' with the consequences, rock beats scissors (blunts them), scissors beats paper (obviously) and paper beats rock (yeah I know, this is hard to grasp, but it just is, okay!).

The set-up goes like this. Two people lock eyes upon one another as

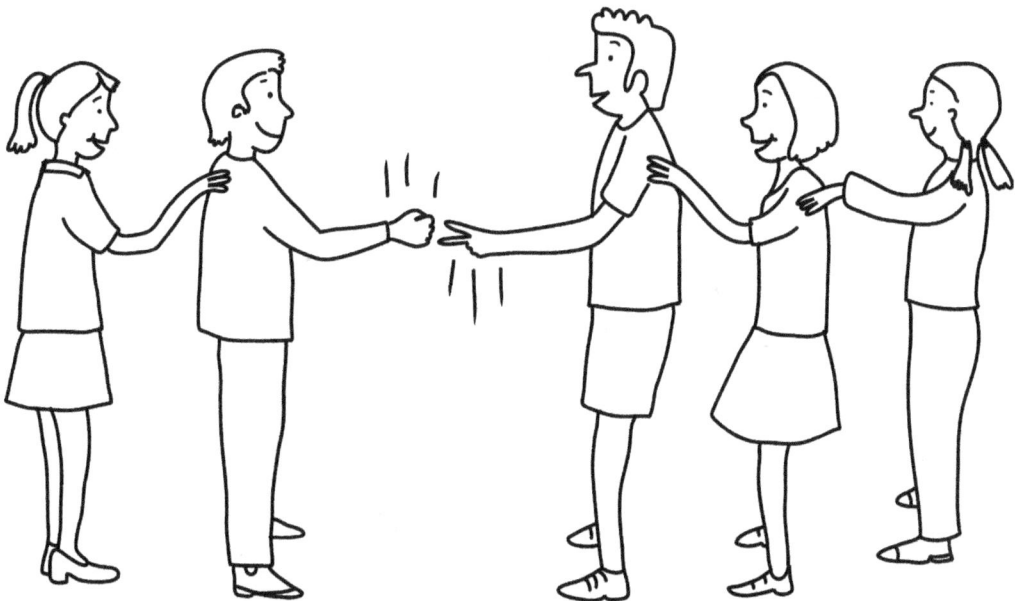

they mingle about the group. They approach, exchange the standard "ONE, TWO, THREE" greeting, and one of them wins. A tie means play again. However, the loser does not in fact 'lose.' He or she joins in the celebrations by following directly behind the 'winner' a la congo-line style. The game continues unabated, with winners winning and losers winning, until there are two giant congo-lines facing off. Upon ushering in the grand winner, wait a few moments for the victors to lick their spoils, and then shout an emphatic "GO," to start it all anew.

Oh, and why 'Ro-Sham-Bo'? – the game is often referred to as such in France and the USA in honour of Jean-Baptiste Donatien de Vimeur, compte de Rochambeau, French hero of American Revolution. Rochambeau was present in York when General Cornwallis surrendered to George Washington. It is believed that Washington, Cornwallis and Rochambeau played 'rock, paper, scissors' to decide who would be the last to leave Cornwallis' tent after the exchange of formalities. At the time, it was considered most honourable to be last. Rochambeau 'won' the game, and it has been known as Ro-Sham-Bo ever since!

Also, did you know that there are professional Ro-Sham-Bo Leagues around the world, and first prize can fetch as much as USD$50,000? I'm in the wrong business!

Variations

- Play this with any game that produces a quick and easy result, such as flipping coins or drawing straws.
- Instruct that the winner of each round 'uses' (that is, plays) the weapon of their most recent opponent in the very next round, to demonstrate that they have won.

TOP MONKEY

A zany game, think 'Simon Says' meets 'ESP'

AT A GLANCE
With their backs initially to a leader, the group turns around on a signal demonstrating one of three animal gestures aiming to match their leader's actions.

WHAT YOU NEED
5 – 10 mins

WHAT TO DO
There are two parts to this ridiculously silly game; the set-up and the play.

To develop the set-up, explain that you are the 'Top Monkey' by making various scratching-under-the-armpit motions like a monkey. Standing in front of you, encourage the crowd to do the same. Tell them that all of the animals in the jungle (them) want to be the Top Monkey. And because she or he (you) is king, the Top Monkey often chooses to imitate the other animals. At this point, decide on three animals you would like to imitate – it doesn't matter which ones you choose, just be sure their actions are unique.

I often go with a racoon (make circles with thumb and pointer fingers on both hands, and peer through them), crocodile (extend both arms out in front, palms facing, and slap together several times) and giraffe (both arms extended above your head, hands clasped and bent forward). With each animal, demonstrate the gesture and ask your group to follow suit. The more animation, the better.

Now for the play. Tell your group that the only way that they can become Top Monkey is by beating Top Monkey at his or her own game, i.e., imitations. With people still facing you, you call "TOP MONKEY" over and over again, each time scratching in all the appropriate spots for good effect. Meanwhile, your group should remain motionless in front of you.

Suddenly, you shout "NOT A MONKEY" which is a trigger for everyone (including you, the Top Monkey) to quickly become one of the three other animals. The trick is that everyone wants to be the same as the animal now revealed by the Top Monkey. Those who match the Top Monkey get to stay in the game, while those who do not, are asked to sit down.

Do the play a few times, so people get the idea. Many people often 'beat' the Top Monkey at this stage, which is good. These trials will build their confidence, just before it really gets interesting.

Announce that you are about to start the game for real, but from now on, everyone will face away from you, the Top Monkey. They turn away, you call out "TOP MONKEY, TOP MONKEY, etc, etc…," during which your group remains motionless. Until you suddenly shout "NOT A MONKEY" as you imitate one of the three animals. Immediately, everyone swings about gesturing their chosen animal as they turn, and voila! Some will be imitating the Top Monkey (hooray), others not (good-bye).

Continue until you are down to the last person, which necessitates a back-to-back showdown in front of everyone. The winner is crowned the new Top Monkey (and handed a banana), and everyone returns for a new game.

Variation

Rather than eliminate people, ask people to keep a record of the number of 'matches' made with Top Monkey. Much like ESP (see page 76).

SLAP HAPPY

Great excuse for a little mayhem whenever you find yourself in a circle

AT A GLANCE

Situated in a circle, each person extends their left hand palm-up and places their right-hand palm down on top of the hand of their right-hand neighbour. On "GO," every person with their palm down attempts to slap the palm-up hand below it as many times as possible.

WHAT YOU NEED

1 – 2 mins

WHAT TO DO

The hardest part of this exercise is the set-up. So let me be very specific.

Start with a circle of people facing into the centre, standing or sitting it doesn't matter. Ask each person to look at their left hand and place it out in front of them, palm facing up. Now, have them look at their right hand (that's the one not being used), and rest it gently palm-down on top of the open palm situated on their right hand side. OK, so far so good.

Now it gets even trickier. The object of the game is for each person to use their right hand (i.e., the one with palm facing down on top of their neighbour's hand) to perform a rapid yet happy little slap (up and down) so that they make contact with their neighbour's hand. Of course, each person is also trying to avoid being 'slapped' by pulling their hand away at the last moment.

It's these twin functions and the delight in making a slap stick that makes this activity so entertaining and incredibly infectious.

A quick word about the slap before I close. While, yes, I do use the word "Slap," I do not mean whack, spank or strike. A simple albeit rapid up and down motion to make contact with a partner's hand is all that is necessary. A blow that produces a red mark is not the aim here.

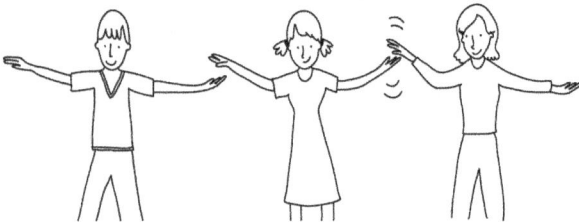

Variations

- Start in pairs first. Same rules apply. Then, as your group becomes accustomed to the highly refined skill of avoiding a back-handed slap, ask two pairs to join and form a quad, and then two quads combine to form an octuplet, and ... well, you get the idea.

- Introduce a rule that when a successful slap occurs, the person with the upward-facing palm switches to become the slap-happy downward facing palm. This is guaranteed to lead to utter mayhem as people often forget which hand is doing what. Perfect.

BUZZ

A timeless, infectious thinking game

AT A GLANCE

Sitting in a circle, a group will count to 100 and beyond – one person giving one number at a time – and substitute any number with the digit or any multiple of seven in it with the word "BUZZ."

WHAT YOU NEED

5 – 10 mins

WHAT TO DO

This is one of those games you either love or hate. I happen to get a kick out of it.

Sit your group down, and explain that you want them to start counting from 1 to 100, perhaps beyond if they are good enough. One person starts with "ONE" and then the person to their left says "TWO" and so on. In response to a number of curious do-you-think-we-are-stupid looks, further explain that for every number that has the digit '7' in it, or is a multiple of seven, the player whose turn is next must substitute the numeral for the word "BUZZ."

So, for example, it will sound like this:

1, 2, 3, 4, 5, 6, **BUZZ**, 8, 9, 10, 11, 12, 13, **BUZZ**, 15, 16, **BUZZ**, 18, 19, …

Get the idea? An old drinking game I'm sure, but alcohol need not wet your lips, because you are sure to intoxicate your group with an intensity of focus and explosive outbursts of laughter that is rarely ever seen.

Idea is, every time a mistake is made in the math, the counting stops, and the group starts over from zero. Work it for five to ten minutes and see how far they get.

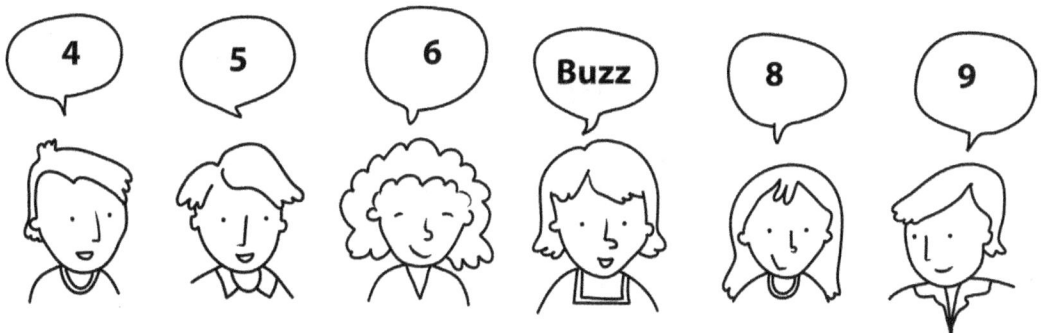

Variation

Pick another number to substitute, for example, '3.' Works best with odd numbers.

PDQ TEST

One of the silliest, most bizarre invitations to have FUNN

AT A GLANCE
A series of dexterous hand, face and body manipulations presented one at a time to a group, inviting them to copy and perhaps present their own.

WHAT YOU NEED
2 – 10 mins

WHAT TO DO
You can never have enough activities that fill in idle time, and this is one of the best. First presented to me by Karl Rohnke – he of the rubbery face and double-jointed limbs – I proudly add to his efforts, and introduce the PDQ or Play Determined Quotient Test. As you will see, it's not so much a test as it is an invitation to play.

Gather your folks, and invite them to sit down, catch their breath, wait, whatever the intent of their idleness. Announce that you are going to introduce a 'Test.' As you proceed, indicate that only each individual will be aware of their own score – you either pass or fail at each level. Also explain that the test will build in its complexity. At this juncture, directly before I start the test, I also point out that this is MY Test, because, as my group will soon witness, I can pass all parts of it.

To begin. Here is a common sequence I use to introduce my PDQ Test. You have a few of your own physical concoctions to present – knock yourself out!

1. Click your fingers. Most people will immediately turn to their dominant hands and fingers. So, invite everyone to use their less-dominant hand now, and then on both hands, click with their less dominant-fingers.

2. Whistle. It's amazing, but not everyone can do this. I always joke around here, and suggest that if you can't whistle, just sit or stand a little closer to someone who can and make a whistle-like mouth, so that if anyone were watching you, they'd think you could!!

3. Cheek Popping. Poke your extended pointer finger inside your mouth and against the inside of your cheek (keeping your lips pursed) and quickly snap it forward and out of the mouth to create that familiar "POP" sound. Try both sides of your cheek. Try it with less dominant fingers.

4. Wiggle Waggle. I did say it would get more difficult with time, and I'm just referring to me writing the description. With hands pressed against each other as in a prayer, slide the middle finger of each hand past the other so that it bends and sticks out past the rest of the upright fingers. Now, carefully slide your palms and remaining fingers so that they end up resting 180 degrees from where they started. If you did this correctly, you should have your two middle fingers juxtaposed one another wiggle waggling to the top and bottom of your down and up-turned palms. If not, you may have broken a finger!!

5. Whistle into your hands. Clasp your hands together so that one hand

cups neatly and water-tightly into the cup of the other. You should aim to have your two thumbs resting side by side, with a slim opening between them. Hold this empty vessel directly against your bottom lip (or there abouts – it's slightly different for each person), blow across the top of the opening between your thumbs, and create a wonderful hollow whistling sound. It's similar to what you can achieve blowing across the top of an open glass drink bottle.

6. Finger Sausages. Bring your two clenched hands in front of you, and extend the two index fingers so that they touch. Now, look at the point at which these fingers touch, and notice the linked sausage. See it? If you can't, try looking beyond your fingers (and not at them), and the linked sausage will suddenly jump out at you. Feeling hungry, try all fingers touching in front of you. Wow – four linked sausages! Now for the best part – pull your fingers away from each other slightly, and voila! Observe a rack of floating human finger sausages!!

7. Tongue Twisters. Poke out your tongue and curl it so that it looks a bit like the letter U. Can you do it the other way, i.e., an upside down U? I can't, so therefore it's not part of my test. Can you touch your nose with your tongue? That I can do.

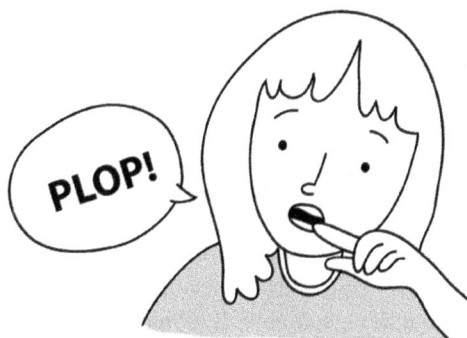

8. Touch your hands behind your back. Take one hand and place it behind your back over your shoulder, while extending the otherhand around your side so that it touches your other hand.

And the list could go on. Every group that I have introduced this activity to has willingly volunteered one or more other tests. Wiggling ear-lobes, flaring nostrils, thumbs that can bend all the way back to the wrist, playing a tune with air emitted from an arm-pit cavity, etc. They're often all the things that we got in trouble for at school when we were caught impressing our friends in the back row!

The most bizarre manipulations I have ever witnessed? I'll share two with you. A guy who, with his right palm pressed firmly onto the floor, could twist his arm (and body) 540 degrees without his palm moving. Or, what about the woman who could put her whole clenched fist into her mouth. Yahhhhhhhh.

Variation

Having first introduced a few simple PDQs of your own, ask a number of small groups to discover a few of their own, and challenge other groups to try them out.

DOWN BY THE BANKS

One of the squillions of hand-clapping games out there

AT A GLANCE

Standing in a circle, and having placed their right hands on top of their neighbours' left hands, everyone slaps hands from right to left one at a time as they sing a little ditty until, on the final beat, someone is eliminated.

WHAT YOU NEED

5 – 10 mins

WHAT TO DO

Start with a circle of not more than 10 to 15 people. With large groups, even better (you'll see why in a moment), create several small circles of people. Choosing one group to demonstrate, ask everyone to find a vantage point and watch and listen closely.

Standing as part of a circle facing in, ask each person to hold out their left hand, palms facing up. Then, ask everyone to place their right hands, palm facing up on top of their neighbour's left hand.

Next, explain that with each beat of a little ditty you will soon teach them, one person at a time will slap their right hand (arcing right to left) into the up-turned hand of their left-hand side neighbour (which of course is resting atop of their left hand). So it goes – beat (slap), beat (slap), beat (slap),

and so on. Of course, while I say slap, I do not mean to leave a red raw brand. A simple light pat is fine.

Having been around the block a few times, I'm sure there are a ton of alternative lyrics for this little ditty, but no matter. It's all about having fun, or is that, FUNN? Here are the lyrics as I was taught many moons ago (X = slap):

DOWN (X) BY THE BANKS (X) OF THE HANKY (X) PANKY (X)
WHERE THE BULL (X) FROG JUMPS (X) FROM THE BANK (X) TO BANKY (X)
SINGING EEEPS (X), IIIPS (X), OOOPS (X), UUUPS (X)
KNEE-SUCKER (X) DILLY DALLY (X) DING (X), DANG (X), DONG (X)

It doesn't take long for the group to catch onto the lyrics. Practice it a few times, working hard to maintain the rhythm of the beat.

The idea is to not be the 'DONG,' i.e., the person who has their hand slapped on this final word. If you are the DONG, you are politely asked to leave the circle, and the game resumes with the person to the Donger's left. Action continues until there are two final people, at which point, a quick game of 'rock-paper-scissors' does the trick.

Variation

When working with a large group (i.e., you have lots of small groups operating), ask all those who are eliminated to form a new circle. You'll find new circles starting up all the time. That's good. When the energy wanes, it's time to move on.

DO AS I SAY

A deceptively simple, yet clever twist of a 'golden-oldie'

AT A GLANCE

One at a time, people perform a simple action while saying that they are doing something quite different, to cue the next person in turn to perform what the first person just said, while saying something else.

WHAT YOU NEED

5 – 10 mins

WHAT TO DO

Here's another classic 'follow me' exercise that I always seem to mess up. I guess that's why it's so much fun.

You could involve your whole large group in one big circle, but I've found that that lacks intimacy, so I suggest separating your group into smaller groups of, say, 10 to 15 people. Demonstrate what needs to happen before splitting up though.

You start by inviting a couple of volunteers to join you in a straight line facing your group. Then, you say "I LIKE TO JUMP UP AND DOWN," but, you are, in fact doing something quite different, perhaps waving your arms up and down. In other words, you are actually DOing something completely different from what you SAY you like to do.

Next, the person to your left will actually do what you said you like doing, but say they like something else. For example, this second person will jump up and down (to copy what I said), but will say that they like something else, such as "I like to ride horses." The next person makes like riding a horse, and so on... In essence, each person DOES what they heard the person before them say, while saying that they like to do something quite different and unique.

The aim of the game is to work your way around the circle and avoid making mistakes. Accuracy is the key, but for your high performance groups, I suggest that pace and unique actions are also key success factors. So, if someone should pause to think too long, or repeat an action someone has already performed, the game stops. Oh, the squeals of laughter...

On most occasions, I don't bother to eliminate people, but you could of course head in this direction until you are left with an eventual 'winner.'

Variations

- As an added getting-to-know-you bonus, make it a group goal to remember the 'like' action of each person.

- Rather than saying and doing a series of actions, each person simply points to a particular part of their body but in doing so names it as another part of their body. For example, I may say "THIS IS MY NOSE" but I actually point at my elbow. The next person will then point at their nose but say "THIS IS MY ELBOW" and follow with "THIS IS MY KNEE" but actually point somewhere else. Basically, each person copies the opposite of what the person before them said and did. Get it? Yeah, I know, it does my head in too.

PEOPLE TO PEOPLE TWISTER

A twisted variation of the popular 'People to People' activity

AT A GLANCE

Standing back to back in pairs, people make contact with matching parts of their partner's body in response to a series of calls from a leader.

WHAT YOU NEED

5 – 10 mins

WHAT TO DO

Divide your group into pairs and ask them to stand back to back. Everyone needs a partner, plus one left over – hopefully you. To whet your group's appetite for what is about to take place, provoke an image in their minds about the fantastic 70s game of 'Twister.' You know, "Left hand on blue," and "Right knee on yellow."

Next, explain that you will soon announce a series of anatomical parts of the human body which will be each person's cue to touch the matching part of their partner. So, if you say "HEAD TO HEAD," each person will gently move their head to touch the head of their partner. Or, if you say "LEFT FOOT TO BACK OF RIGHT KNEE," each person will take their left foot to touch the back of their partner's right knee. Remember, all of this is done standing back to back. Got it?

Naturally, there is always a line that can be crossed here, and it's obvious to most people, but you are well advised to frame your introduction to frown upon inappropriate calls.

Anyway, this friendly twisted anatomical shuffle continues until the person holding the floor decides they have had enough, or can't think of any more parts of the human body, and calls out "PEOPLE TO PEOPLE." On this cue, everyone is requested to find a new partner. The person making the call joins

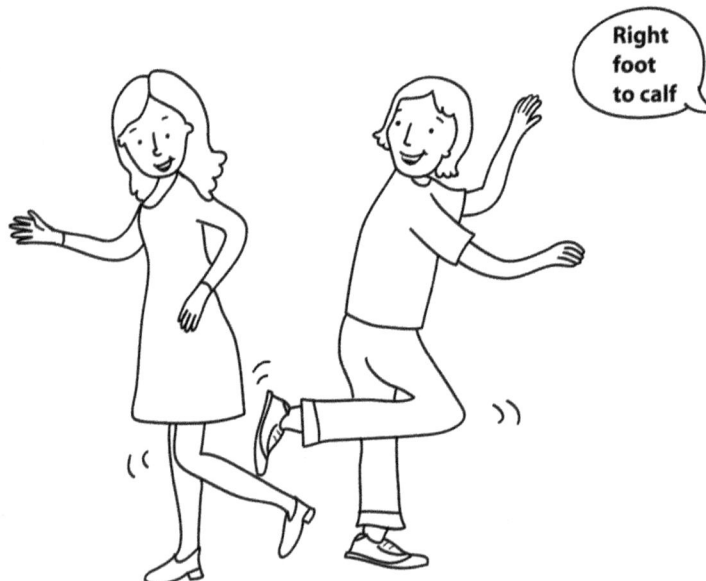

Right foot to calf

in the search for partnership, and eventually, you're left with a new leader.

Note: as part of my briefing, I always explain what to do if someone finds themselves 'in the middle' by offering them an out. There's an obvious one here – they simply call the words "PEOPLE TO PEOPLE" – but, in other games, I suggest they simply say "HEY, WHO WANTS TO SWAP WITH ME?" and someone is always, always willing to steal the limelight.

Variations

- Pairs face one another, clap to a slow beat, and then upon the call, touch their partner's matching body part with their own twice while also repeating the call, e.g., "HAND TO CHEEK. (a beat) HAND TO CHEEK."

- In groups of four to six people, one person elects to become the anatomical magnet for his or her mates. With each call, one person matches the particular body parts of their partner, until everyone is somehow physically connected to the first person.

TOUCH THAT

Another leaderless activity that provides your group with an opportunity to contribute

AT A GLANCE

People move about a pre-defined area and respond immediately to the call of anyone from the group to touch something, and then, upon everyone accomplishing this task, resume their walk.

WHAT YOU NEED

5 – 10 mins

WHAT TO DO

When it comes to touching, OK, I know what you're thinking. This activity could be a disaster if not presented appropriately. So, I can not emphasise strongly enough the capacity of your sequencing and framing to influence the value and thus result of this activity.

That said, this is what you do (which is not much). Invite your group to position themselves evenly throughout some pre-defined area, and upon the command "WALK," ask everyone to just mill about the area. No touching, no talking, just walking.

Then, at any time, any person may choose to call out a command to touch something, such as "TOUCH BLACK." This will instruct everyone to immediately find some object that is black and touch it. What is doing the touching is not important, so long as some part of the anatomy is physically connected to the said thing. Once everyone is touching the aforementioned object, a new person is able to call "WALK." A few moments later, another person calls out "TOUCH AN ELBOW," and so the action continues.

Even with the best of intentions, your group may be tempted to enter the nether regions or simply ask their group to touch or do something that will make them uncomfortable. To this end, I always preface the first "WALK" with something like this:

"...Think carefully about what you're going to ask others to do before you say it. Remember, the idea is to create a fun and supportive environment, and not make it hard for others. And I don't just mean asking others to touch certain parts of the body that some people won't want to have touched. Asking people to perform a back-flip while holding their breath is just as uncomfortable...."

As with Stop & Go (page 92), how you stop the game is up to you. Either just step in and say, "OK, that's enough," or suggest that whenever five or more people remain touching the most recent 'thing' after the call to move has been given, the game is over.

Variations

- Invite group members to nominate the way in which people move about the area, rather than walk. "WALK BACKWARDS," "HOP ON ONE FOOT," and "SLOW MOTION" are all good examples.

- One way to escalate the energy is to move from one thing to another with simultaneous commands, such as "TOUCH DENIM & HOP," or "TOUCH WOOD & HOLD YOUR BREATH." For a bit of fun, call out "TOUCH SHOULDERS & MASSAGE."

- To add to the challenge, explain that in the process of obtaining the 'touch,' no one is permitted to touch anyone else.

DOG SHAKE

Permission to act like a dog for just a minute, granted

AT A GLANCE

Following the lead of another, a person will gyrate their body as if they were a dog shaking itself after getting wet.

WHAT YOU NEED

1 – 2 mins

WHAT TO DO

When I first saw Karl Rohnke do this, I could barely contain myself. It's a cack.

Pretty simple. Ask your group to stand in front of you, bunched up works just fine. You start by telling a story about what a dog looks like when it's about to engage in one almighty all-body shake. On all fours (you may choose to do this, but it's not necessary), the body-tremor often starts at the nose. It twitches this way and that, and then the jowls and face get in on the action. Nervous energy then proceeds down the neck as it contorts in and out, when suddenly, the upper torso decides to join in and chunks of flesh just shivers off the rib cage. Now the arms and legs start up, the force of the tremor causing them to perform a shudder never before seen in public when, before you know it, the feet and tail finally come to the party! It's one giant, cataclysmic quiver of body parts and hair. And then it's over. If you've done your pooch proud, you should take a bow.

It's important that you first don a demonstration to inject just the right levels of enthusiasm and silliness into the exercise. Then, it's your group's turn as you exclaim that, "HANG-ON, I FEEL ANOTHER SHAKE COMING ON…"

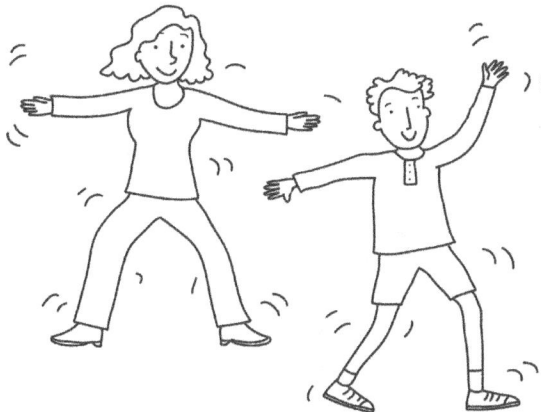

Variations

- Try it again in slow-motion, and then in 'time-warp' speed – top to bottom.
- In pairs, invite one person to perform their best dog shake impersonation, followed by their partner.

EILEEN

Another perfectly silly excuse to kill a minute or two

AT A GLANCE
Standing shoulder to shoulder with others in a circle, people slowly lean into the circle aiming to support everyone's weight for as long as possible.

WHAT YOU NEED
1 – 2 mins

WHAT TO DO
How often in a program do you ask your group to form a circle? Well, add one more to the count. But this time, ask everyone to form as perfect a circle as possible. No bends, no corners, just a perfectly round-edged circle. Good, now come in closer, and closer still – until everyone is just touching the shoulders of their neighbours. Stop there.

Your next move is to invite everyone to lean in slowly. And as they produce moderate levels of balance and comfort, to slowly, ever so slowly, edge their feet backwards just a smidge or two. The goal is to create what's called a 'yurt' – an engineering term to describe a self-supporting structure. Or, at least that's what I know it as! Keep this up for as long as possible.

With each smidgen, review the balance and composure of your group, and if considered safe, suggest stepping back a little further. Anything up to 30cm (1') extended back from the starting position is cool; beyond this point, encourage your group to brace for a topple, or be ready to stop the exercise.

There's something pretty special about a large group of people leaning in toward each other attempting to reach that pinnacle of balance, where just one bad move will cause the pieces to topple just like a string of dominos. It rarely happens, but that's not the point, is it?

Although it seems obvious, it is always a good idea to remind people that they should take a step forward if they feel that they are going to fall.

Oh, and by the way. Eileen? Get it?

Variation

Ever mindful of your sequence and the safety considerations of your group, try it backwards, asking your participants to face out of the circle. Often works a little better because we tend to have more beefy edges to the back of our shoulders than the front. Well, I do anyway.

DEPORTMENT TAG

A fun variation of tag that encourages good posture

AT A GLANCE

On "GO," everyone moves about an area stiffly, attempting to tag other people without touching or dropping the small objects that are perched on their heads.

WHAT YOU NEED

A small object for each person, e.g., eraser, pencil, bean-bag toy, etc

2 – 5 mins

WHAT TO DO

Good deportment teaches proper posture. So does this game of tag.

First, ask everyone to find a small inanimate object, such as an eraser, bean-bag toy, pen or pencil. To avoid those nagging comments of "That's not fair, his is smaller / lighter / stickier than mine," it works best if everyone can use the same type of object.

Then, resting the object on top of one's head, the action starts. Everyone is 'It' and attempts to tag as many people as possible while trying to avoid being tagged. If at anytime someone feels the urge to touch their object to arrest its fall, or their item does fall, they are eliminated. Game continues until one perfectly postured player remains.

If the action evaporates too quickly, suggest that everyone has three lives before they are eliminated.

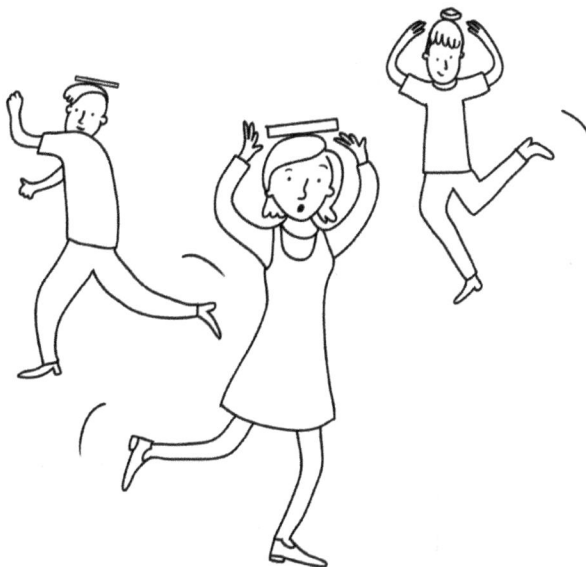

Variations

- To effect a successful tag, a person must 'steal' the object on his or her opponent's head. This will cause all manner of avoidance strategies which invariably end up with an item on the ground. To prolong the action, have each person balance two or three items on their head, giving them two or three lives, so to speak.

- Try any of your favourite tag games with a sophisticated level of deportment.

KNEE TAG

A popular tag game given a new lease on life

AT A GLANCE

A person standing with his or her hands on his or her knees, attempts to tag the undefended knees of other players as often as possible.

WHAT YOU NEED

5 – 10 mins

WHAT TO DO

Ask everyone to find a partner who has knees that look like theirs. Of course, this is a completely frivolous request, because all you really need are lots of pairs, but observing the brief pursuit of knee comparison is worth it.

Standing with their feet about shoulder-width apart, each person faces their partner about a metre (3') away and bends down slightly to place their hands on their knees. Each combatant eyes the other eagerly and the action begins. A score is made when one person tags the undefended knee of the other, i.e., their partner does not have a hand on that knee for a split second. Naturally, in order to make a tag, a person's hand must vacate their knee, so they are vulnerable to attack as well.

Mr or Ms Smarty-pants will think that if they never take their hands off their knees they can't lose. Perhaps. But what a boring way to live your life – which is what we're talking about here, right?

Safety note – watch your head. The focus is all on the knees and hands, thus there may be a tendency to forget about the possibility of bumping heads as people dart about to prevent being tagged.

Next, look to the variations, because having grasped the basic tenets of this exercise, there is so much more available to you.

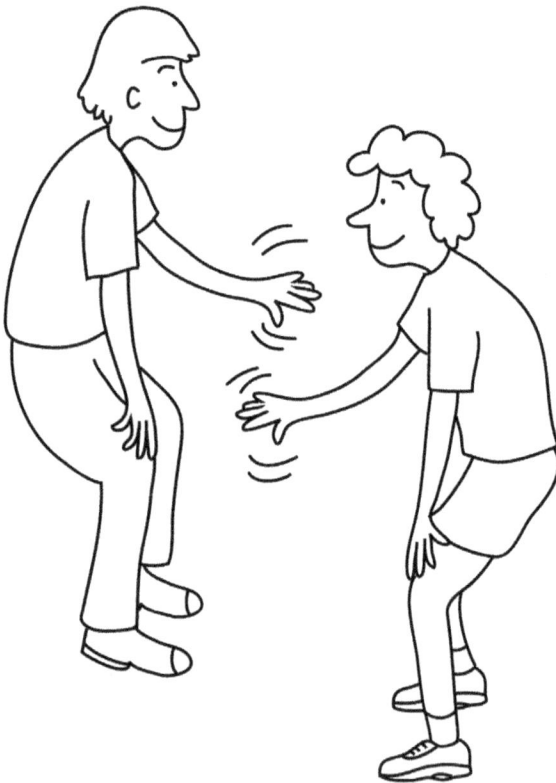

Variations

- Keeping with this same partner, allow people to move from their fixed lead-footed position, perhaps to escape their opponent's reach. However, at all times while their feet are moving, their fingers must be interlocked in front of them. Ah, yes, this means that their knees could be tagged.

- Introduce the ability for people to tag any undefended knees, i.e., those belonging to people moving about them. Remember, all moves (i.e., your feet are moving) must be made with interlocked fingers.

- Introduce the 'HANDS UP' rule. When your group hears you shout, "HANDS UP," everyone must hold their hands up high above their head and not ever defend their knees. They may, of course, choose to lower a hand to make a committed tag of any exposed knees, but that's it! Shortly after, your call of "HANDS DOWN" returns people to the status quo, until the next "HANDS UP" and so on.

BILL & THE BUTTON FACTORY

The craziest 'do-what-I-do' reward for a deserving large group

AT A GLANCE
Your group sings along with a little ditty as they mimic your crazy antics.

WHAT YOU NEED
3 - 5 mins

WHAT TO DO
My strongest recommendation is to pick your moment on this one. Your group has to be 'warmed up,' especially emotionally. You know, there has to be a certain energy in the room, an undeniable willingness to really play and look foolish for a moment or three.

Having decided to reward your group (and having picked your moment), ask them to assemble in front of you, as if they were your audience, because you want to sing a little song about your friend Bill. Really bunch them together. There should be conspicuous interests

being piqued all over the place by now.

Explain that you would like everyone to follow your lead and simply copy everything you say out loud. To test the water, you start with a hearty "HI," and gesture for the crowd to follow suit with a full-bodied "HI." Don't be shy

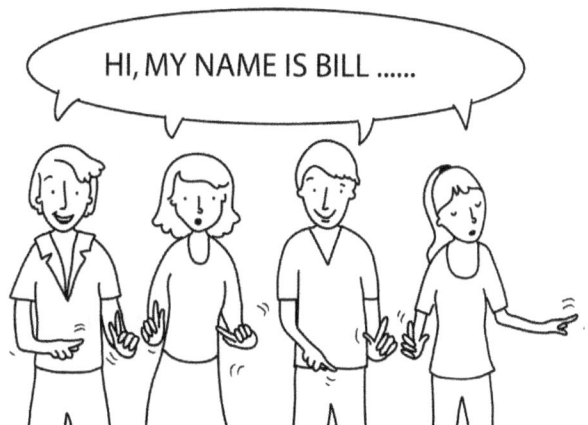

HI, MY NAME IS BILL ......

here – like most things, the success is found in its delivery – the more enthusiasm, conviction and crazy you put into it, the more contagious it becomes.

Having got this 'say-what-I-say' concept, your group is ready to launch into the full ditty. The basic premise is that you say a line, your group repeats the same line directly back at you. Simple. There is a beat, but don't worry too much about that in the beginning. Here are the full lyrics...

"HI.

MY NAME IS BILL.

I HAVE A JOB AND A LIFE IN A BUTTON FACTORY.

ONE DAY.

MY BOSS CAME UP TO ME AND SAID.

HEY BILL.

ARE YOU BUSY?

HECK NO.

THEN PUSH THESE BUTTONS WITH YOUR FINGERS...."

Until the last line, you're simply having fun singing, all the while encouraging your group to emulate your over-the-top enthusiasm and antics. Then the fun begins. Upon singing the "THEN PUSH THESE BUTTONS WITH YOUR FINGERS..." line, you add the committed physical gesture of poking your left and right pointer fingers into the air in front of you as if you were pressing a series of buttons on a machine – all the time, keeping to a beat (I like to alternate the fingers, e.g., left, right, left, right...), and encouraging your group to follow suit.

Now, continue with the finger poking, and within a few moments start over with "HI" (the group responds) and you repeat the whole verse again (all the time, foolishly poking the air), until the last line when you add more buttons to be pressed. But with each verse, you choose a unique part of the anatomy to do its share of the poking. Here are my favourite suggestions...

"THEN PUSH THESE BUTTONS WITH YOUR ELBOWS..." (you now poke alternately with fingers and elbows)

"THEN PUSH THESE BUTTONS WITH YOUR KNEES..." (fingers, elbows and knees at same time)

"THEN PUSH THESE BUTTONS WITH YOUR TONGUE...." (adding to above actions, it is heart-stopping hilarious).

I find that after four verses, often finishing with "...YOUR TONGUE," I am ready to complete a final passionate, albeit garbled, final verse ending with...

... ARE YOU BUSY (Are you busy?)
HECK YEAH!!

And that's it. The group will often be falling about the floor in fits of laughter – most of it directed at you!

Variation

Make up your own little ditty and / or actions. Perhaps the lyrics or actions relate to a role or favourite person in your organisation? Only one rule – make it FUNN.

PRIMAL SCREAM

An utterly wacky way to release a lot of energy quickly

AT A GLANCE

From a standing line-up, a group of people run full pelt and scream as loudly as they can until they run out of breath.

WHAT YOU NEED

A lot of gumption
1 minute

WHAT TO DO

It was hot, we were all tired, and the sun was dipping behind the trees. Enter, Karl Rohnke. In his mind, the time was just right for one final burst of energy. Karl introduced this totally bizarre activity (in which I was a participant) many, many years ago, and I still scratch my head for answers. But it works, really works.

As you will soon understand, you have to pick your moment. Once picked, ask your group to kind of line up at one end of a large hall, playing field or other wide expanse, and point to the other end as the ultimate goal. If you find yourself in a small area, have your group go there and back, or run the perimeter.

The object, you will explain, is to reach that other end as quickly as possible, but with two provisos. One, the distance must be spanned in one breath, and two, each person will scream at the top of their lungs – any thing they like – as long as it's loud. Basically, you contend that everyone should just run and scream for as long as they have breath left in their lungs. Stop – or collapse as the case may be – once the breath has expired.

Okay, I know it's crazy, but it is totally cool being a part of this extraordinary display of energy...and an even more remarkable spectacle just watching it. So, take a deep breath, and... "GO! ARRRGGGHHHHHHH...."

Word of warning: If you spot any unsuspecting people within ear shot of your assault, re-consider your options.

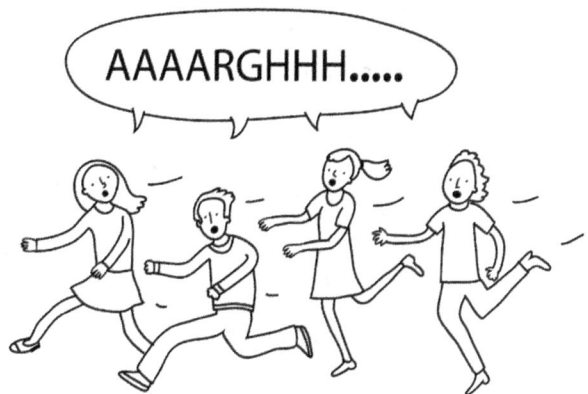

Variation

Same as above, but invite people to scream a few choice words and phrases that would represent their enjoyment or otherwise of a particular activity. A debrief of sorts.

NAME GAMES

Here are a bunch of ideas that I have found encourage and enable people to learn one another's names. Yeah, I know it's hard with large numbers of people, but the higher the level of name-knowingness, the more fun (and trust) your group will develop.

The name-games I describe here feature:

- Fun and laughter as a vital ingredient
- Emphasis on effort, rather than results
- Opportunities to reinforce a cooperative and supportive environment
- 2 to 15 minutes of play

Chunk It

Most people, if they were being honest, would admit that learning names can be hard at times. This being the case, starting with one large (read, overwhelming) group can be problematic. I recommend 'chunks.' Separate your group into smaller units, or 'chunks' perhaps later combining smaller groups to form progressively larger groups. This approach heightens the quality of interaction along the journey, not to mention the fun and ability for people to learn incrementally.

As an example, start by introducing your chosen activity to a series of smaller groups, then swap half of one group with another group. Do this several times, and then slowly combine the groups until eventually you have one massive group.

Presented in a sequence generally reflecting an increasing level of difficulty, here are my favourite name-games. Enjoy!

Name-Tag Mania
Let Me Introduce
Me You You Me
Toss-A-Name-Game
ID Crisis
Kram Dralloc
Partner Introductions
Alpha Line Up
Name Roulette
Who Is It?
Bumpity Bump Bump Bump
Motion Name-Game
Concentration
Peek-A-Who
Cocktail Party

NAME-TAG MANIA

A creative adjunct to many other name-game, mixing activities

AT A GLANCE
Wearing a colourful name-tag that they have drawn, each person will meet and greet other members of their group and share the significance of what is drawn on their tag.

WHAT YOU NEED
Blank name-tag for each person
Coloured markers / pens to share
10 – 20 mins

WHAT TO DO
You are about to ask your group to be creative. Some will drop their shoulders as a result, but I am always amazed at the results – I'm sure you will be too. Integrate elements of this exercise with some of your favourite mixing, getting-to-know-you games.

Distribute a blank name-tag to everyone, or other small blank card with suitable pinning device. With a large box of coloured markers and pens available to everyone, ask each person to write their name in large letters in the top half of the name-tag / card, and then stop. Next, ask everyone to draw three or four objects under their name, which typically represent something about who they are.

Naturally, sky's the limit, but I regularly ask people to draw objects that represent things such as where they live, their occupation, their home, something about their family, favourite pastimes, etc. There are no wrong answers here.

After a few minutes, and having pried the pens from the hands of the terminally creative, ask everyone to pin their name-tag onto their chests, and they're good to go. The goal – to meet and greet as many people as they can in five or so minutes. To my way of thinking, the simple fact that people are invited to focus on the tags, and not the other person (as such), is one reason that this activity works so well. It's less threatening, and, oh, people just love looking at other people's drawings!

There are literally dozens of interactive ways to make use of these artistically inspired tags. All involve a simple sharing of names and the significance (or otherwise) of the drawn objects. Try the following:

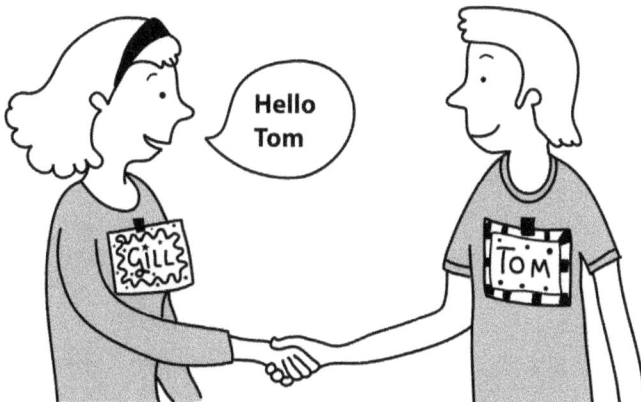

Variations

- Use a variety of groupings (see Categories on page 45) to invite people to find others of a similar ilk. For example, those who used the same colour marker to write their name, those who exclusively used capitals / lower case / mix of letters, those who drew a similar type of first object (e.g., animal, building, person, activity, etc), the number of colours used on the tag, etc.
- Use differently coloured paper to create your name-tags, to nominate colour as another 'category' to divide your group.
- Frame the type of objects you wish to have drawn on the name-tags. For example, draw three of your favourite foods, or sports, or garments of clothing, or – even tougher – personal values.

LET ME INTRODUCE

An exercise where you introduce everyone but yourself

AT A GLANCE

Each person approaches as many people as possible within a specified time limit, introducing each of them to another person in the group.

WHAT YOU NEED

2 – 5 mins

WHAT TO DO

I've found this simple re-working of the traditional form of introductions a brilliant way to rid my group of a lot of that tension that most people experience when they first get together. It won't evaporate all of the awkward feelings, but it is fun and is guaranteed to create a ton of energy.

With your group milling about, ask them to casually approach any other person in the group – whether they know their name or not – greet them, and ask for their name. Embodied with a lively demonstration, it will sound something like this. "HI, WHAT'S YOUR NAME?" The doe-eyed person you have just approached says "SIMON," and you reply with "HI SIMON, COME WITH ME, I'D LIKE TO YOU TO MEET SOMEBODY." At which point you lead Simon to another unsuspecting group member, and say "HI, WHAT'S YOUR NAME?" and it might be Vijay this time. "HI VIJAY. I'D LIKE YOU TO MEET SIMON. SIMON THIS IS VIJAY."

Having done the job of the Introducer, explain that each person now moves on to either seek a new person to greet, or submit to another person's invitation to be part of their introduction, and so on. Get the idea?

In principle, the person arranging the introductions need not say their name, but we are so accustomed to doing so in our culture, it often happens anyway!

To give the exercise a little vivacity, announce that your group has three (or whatever) minutes to introduce everyone to everybody else. Won't happen, but that's not the point.

Variation

Following on from the basic set-up, one of the two people who have just been introduced to each other now leads the other to a new person. For example, Simon leads Vijay over to meet and greet with Rachel.

ME YOU YOU ME

A know-your-own-name-game classic in the making

AT A GLANCE

Walking around the inside of a circle, each person introduces his or her name and repeats the name of every other person in a particular sequence one at a time.

WHAT YOU NEED

5 - 10 mins

WHAT TO DO

This is a great example of an activity once deemed suitable for small groups only, but now has a new lease on life. I'll start with the original set-up, and then describe its application for large groups.

Start with a circle of at least 10 and up to 20 people. Using your example as a demonstration, step in front of the person who was standing to your left. Shake this person's hand, and simply say your own name. Nothing else, no "How do you do," or "My name is...," simply state your name. Whilst still shaking hands, your partner will now say his or her name. Pretty easy so far, but it's not over. Here comes the hard part.

The person who first introduced him or her self (you in the case of this demonstration), now repeats back the name of the person they are greeting (you're still shaking hands by the way). Again, nothing more, just repeat their name. And your partner repeats your name back to you. Phew, it's over, you can unclasp sweaty hands, and move on to the next person, to your right in the circle. So, if I were starting, and your name was Ruby, our exchange would sound like this – "MARK," "RUBY," "RUBY," "MARK."

The process continues with each greeter moving to his or her right (on the inside of the circle), allowing the person next in line to fall in behind them to greet the person the first greeter has just greeted – just like a snake, get it? Each person will walk on the inside of the circle and greet everyone once, and then resume their original position in the circle, and then have every other person greet them

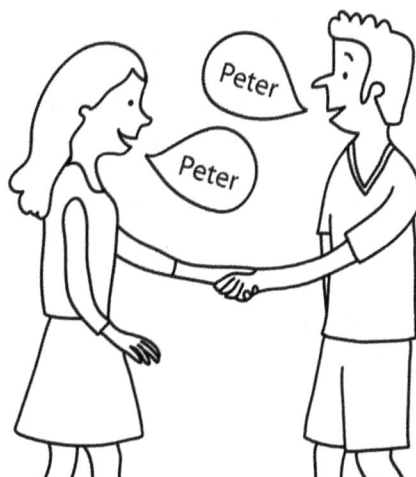

a second time as these folks return to their original spot.

It really is very simple. It's just not easy. And I can almost guarantee you, inside the time it takes for the first few exchanges to occur, the group will erupt in guffaws as one or more people mix up their names. It's astonishing how often people 'use' the wrong name at the wrong time. Ahh, reminds me of many awkward social situations. Anyway...

So, what do you with a large group of say 50, or 100 people? Well, you can split this number into several smaller groups (and follow as above), but if you want to keep them all together, peel off from two or more directions at the same time. So, you get one 'snake' started off to your left, and then after a few exchanges, leave the head of that snake and start a new one on the right hand side of the circle from whence you were standing. The two or more snakes will eventually collide, and confusion will reign. But that's OK, some groups will persist to make it work, others will just look to you and say "HELP!" Just smile.

Now, if you thought this was all about learning names, you've missed the point. Yes, some may pick up a few names, but it's all about taking subtle risks, sharing and above all, laughing.

Variation

Exchange the use of a name with something interesting about yourself, e.g., honest, fun, thirty-two, Brazilian, etc. That was not meant to sound like a personal ad, but you get the idea. So, it may sound like "BUFFED," "FINNISH," "FINNISH," "BUFFED."

ID CRISIS

It's 'Chinese Whispers' meets 'Partner Introductions'

AT A GLANCE

Each person will meet and greet as many people as possible, sharing particular information about themselves with their partners, and then swap name-tags and each assume the identity of the other person as they partake in their next exchange.

WHAT YOU NEED

Small index card, or name-tag, and pen for each person
10 – 20 mins

WHAT TO DO

If your group does not already have individual name-tags, start by distributing a set of index cards and pens and ask everyone to write their names really big on a card.

Next, invite each person to think of their response to a number of specific questions. For example, you could ask each person to think of:

- Their favourite movie;
- The most enjoyable aspect of their occupation or study; and
- What they would do if they won the lottery.

Having absorbed this information, ask everyone to start mingling and greet one other person. If you have an odd number, a group of three works fine. Explain that you would like each pair to get to know one another by sharing anything that is of interest, but at a minimum, they must cover the responses to the three questions you announced. Encourage each person to pay particular attention to these three bits of information about their partner. No need to say anymore just yet.

Allow a minute or two to pass, then halt the conversation and explain that you would now like each person to swap their 'name-tag' with their partner. And – here's the fun bit – each person will now assume the identity of their partner, and share only those three bits of information they learned about their partner, plus anything else they have cared to remember. After a few groans and feverish re-checking of data, the process resumes, but this time, people will be standing in for their most recent partners.

Permit the banter to flow for 10 minutes or so, inviting each person to complete as many exchanges as possible. By now, everyone is thoroughly confused as to who they are. Circle up, and ask one person to start the naming process by 'introducing' themselves, using only the information they can recall about the person named on the tag that they are presently holding. People rarely get it 100% right, so there's always a lot of laughter as the 'real' person identifies him or herself and reworks the data. This person goes next, introducing him or herself as the person named on the name-tag, and so on.

It sometimes occurs that an individual will receive their own 'name-tag' back during the whirl of greetings. That's okay, but they need to take note of the new data about themselves, and not revert back to their original declaration.

Variation

If memory-recall is an issue, allow the original partners to write down their three (or more) bits of information about themselves on the back of the 'tag.' Exchanges proceed as per normal, but this time, people have a crutch to lean on.

TOSS-A-NAME-GAME

An all-time classic name-game, with a few new twists

AT A GLANCE
People stand in a circle passing soft tossable items to each other as they call and learn each other's names.

WHAT YOU NEED
Bunch of soft tossable items
10 – 20 mins

WHAT TO DO
Got a really large group? No trouble – follow the 'chunking' advice at the start of this section. I've worked this classic name-game very successfully with groups of up to 80 people!

To start, ask your group to form a square without sides, and pull a soft

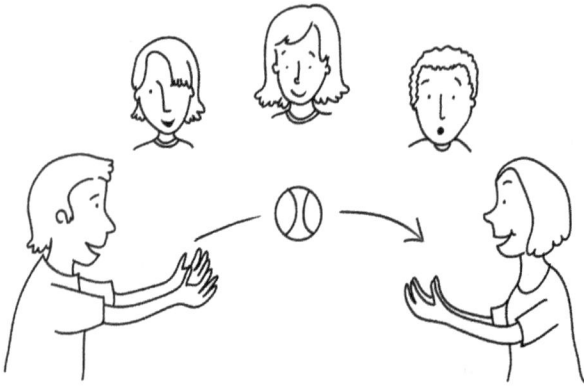

tossable from your pocket, such as a fleece-ball, koosh or beanie baby. Explain that this tossable has been known to possess special name-remembering qualities, and you would like to pass this magic around.

Begin by passing it from left to right around the circle, asking that each person simply say their name (loudly enough for everyone to hear) as they receive it. This may be the first time the group has heard everyone's names. Upon returning to you, pass the tossable back the other way, and repeat the process, but this time ask that everyone remembers at least one other person's name before it gets back you.

Now the fun begins. Whoever has the tossable is now entitled to pass it (notice I said "pass," and not zing!!) to

anyone in the circle, but must first call that person's name. Their attention is attracted, they anxiously await the toss, and voila! it's received. Nice pass. The process continues.

At some point, as the general level of name-knowingness increases, secretly introduce a second tossable into the mix. Notice the discernable groans of anguish as the group acknowledges what has just occurred. Keep adding extra tossables, each one initiating a new exchange of names. Chaos will hold sway, but don't worry too much. People will be having fun, and learning names in the process.

To further reinforce names, ask the people who receive an item to say "THANK YOU" to the person who tossed it to them, but most importantly, using that person's name. Yes, this is trickier, because the receiver has no control over who passes to them. Ideal for encouraging a helpful "SORRY, WHAT IS YOUR NAME?" exchange.

Eventually, after five, ten or more minutes, throw down the gauntlet and challenge one or more folks to name as many people in the group as possible (notice, I didn't say "name everyone"). No matter how big the group is, there is always one person who will give it a go.

Variations

- An ideal twist for folks who have trouble remembering names – interrupt the game, and revert to one tossable again. This time, the tosser will aim to attract eye contact of the person to whom they wish to pass, but does not call his or her name. Instead, as the person receives the pass, everyone in the circle calls out the receiver's name. That's right! A player could deliberately pass the item to someone he or she doesn't know – brilliant. Repeat for a minute or two, then revert back to the original play.

- Once several tossables have been introduced, and with ample space, ask people to take one step back out of the circle when they receive an item. A minute or two later, ask that they take one step back in.

- Suggest that the tossable is no longer a ball – invite your group to imagine that it has turned into something else, a watermelon, perchance. So, from now on, all future passes will reflect the weight and size of a watermelon, or whatever object it is deemed to be. A little later, introduce a second tossable, this time a shot-put, then a feather, then a shoe, etc.

KRAM DRALLOC

A name-game that makes everyone sound wonderfully exotic

AT A GLANCE

One at a time, each person will recite their name backwards to the group.

WHAT YOU NEED

2 – 5 mins

WHAT TO DO

Names are endlessly fascinating, and there's no shortage of silly little games that can be made of them. Here's one to get you started, and then try one or more of the variations.

Ask everyone – one at a time – to say their name out loud as if the letters of their names were arranged in reverse. So, Mark Collard, becomes Kram Dralloc. Get it? Ok, your turn Nasus, then Gerg.

For a little more fun, ask your group to postulate which part of the world, perhaps country or town, this strange sounding name could originate. I reckon mine was coined somewhere in Copenhagen, Denmark in the late 18th century. It's amazing how beautifully exotic so many names become once reversed.

The purpose? None other than a good belly laugh.

Variations

- Combine the first letter of your first name with the first two letters of your surname to create a little hyphenated moniker. Said with a little rap music attitude, you can sound very cool, or at least MCo thinks so.

- Separating into small groups to workshop this one, ask each person to invent a nonsensical acronym of their first (or second) name, and then present it to the larger group. For example, KEVIN becomes Kangaroos Eat Vegies In November and MARK could represent Magic Ankle Repair Kit.

- Invite each person, if possible, to share the known meaning behind their name – its literal meaning, or perhaps, the history of how their parents named them. So, Mark? It originates from the Latin god Mars, and my Mum chose this name because she had always liked the name since dating a boy named Mark. Like I said, endlessly fascinating.

PARTNER INTRODUCTIONS

An easy, non-threatening way to get to know who's who in your group

AT A GLANCE

Two people spend some time chatting with each other, seeking prescribed information at a minimum, and then rejoin the larger group to 'introduce' their partner.

WHAT YOU NEED

30 – 40 mins

WHAT TO DO

By the time all of the introductions have occurred, you may not have much change from an hour. But it's worth every minute.

Use a fun method to separate your group into pairs. Shortly, you will invite them to sit down and have a good chat with each other, and in particular, discuss several key getting-to-know-you topics. Here are a few suggestions:

- Their name, where they come from and what they do for a living?

- Their favourite holiday destination?
- The naughtiest thing they ever did as a kid?

Importantly, tell everyone that their goal is to not only share this information (at a minimum), but also to remember what their partner shared. Because, when time's up, each person will be invited to introduce their partner when the large group re-forms. That's right, individuals do not introduce themselves – that's too frightening – they introduce their partners.

After five to ten minutes, gather your group, sit in a circle and commence the introductions. I always seek a volunteer to go first, upon which their partner reciprocates. Then, these two decide who goes next.

You know what they say – the number one fear in the world is speaking in front of others. Well, I have found that when sequenced correctly, this exercise works wonders because – as many shy people often later comment – it's easier when people don't have to speak about themselves. Right there – that's the essence of this activity!

If you have a really large group, i.e., it would take three hours to run through all of the introductions, consider dividing your mob into smaller groups to share.

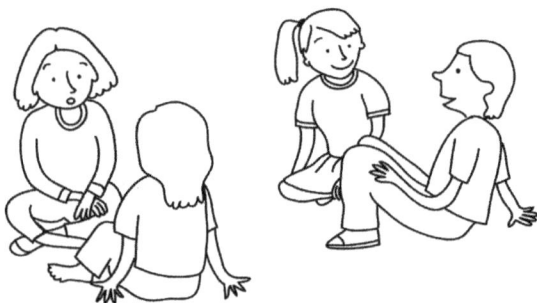

Variations

- Ask the 'introducing' partner to stand behind their subjects as they speak about them.
- Ask the 'introducing' partner to mime their introduction, featuring the three key characteristics of their partner, allowing the rest of the group to guess the answers.

ALPHA LINE UP

A fun, passive exercise on its own, or a great way to segue into other activities

AT A GLANCE

Individuals in a group form one straight line according to the alphabetical order of their first names.

WHAT YOU NEED

2 – 10 mins

WHAT TO DO

Need a line of people to move into your next activity? What about pairs? Well, as a passive activity, this exercise is also a perfect follow-on from more rambunctious activity.

As people are catching their breath, ask them to consider their first name for a moment, and in particular, how it is spelt. Announce next that as a group, their task is to form one straight line according to the alphabetical order of their first names. If two or more people have the same names, use middle and last names to distinguish the order. You may choose to designate where the A and Z are situated, but I often allow the group to work this part out for themselves.

Oh, and by the way, all of this alphabetising is to be performed mute. Yep, that's right, no talking – only non-verbal forms of communication are allowed, e.g., fingers. Once a line is formed, check it for accuracy to help reinforce names. As a problem-solving activity, this is a fantastic exercise for exploring effective communication – so feel free to process the 'goings-on' before you move on.

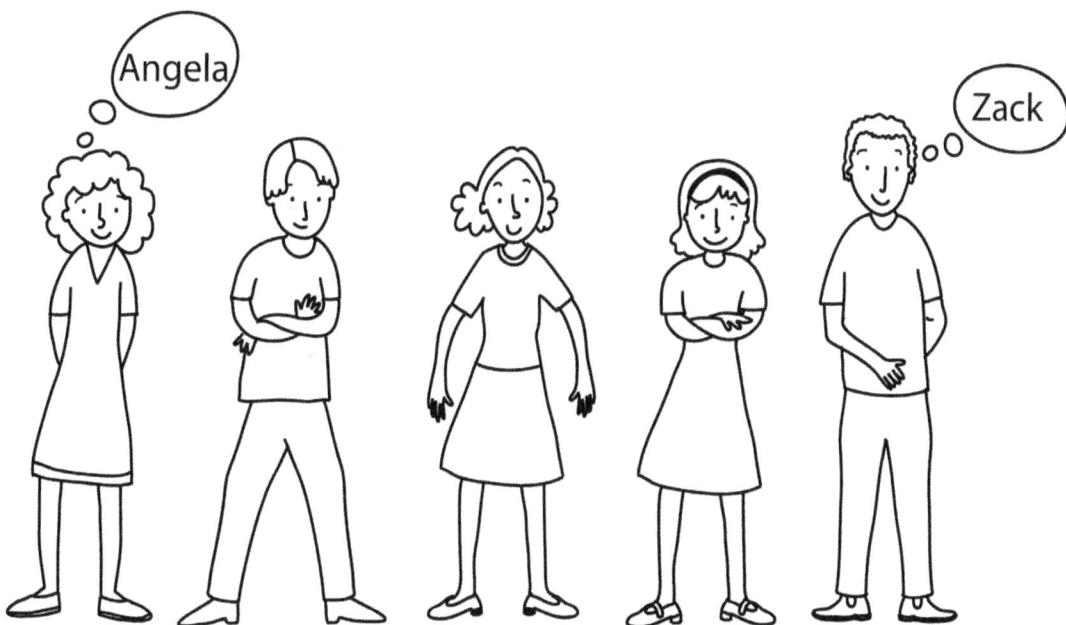

If your program calls for pairs next, fold the line in half so that the person at the far end walks back down the length of the line to stand opposite the person at the start, while the former's fellow line mates follow directly behind to meet their respective partners. Voila! A great way to create random partners.

Variations

- For groups of people who know each other well, use middle names, or some other personal criteria such as:
  - Last two digits of their home phone number
  - Date of their most memorable adventure experience (month and year)
  - Number of their home's street address
  - Birth date (not including the year).
- Ask people to close their eyes (on top of being mute) to make it very difficult.

NAME ROULETTE

A name-reminder game with a casino-esque plot

AT A GLANCE

Two circles of people holding hands rotate directly next to each other. When "STOP" is called, the person from each circle who is closest to a designated spot, will attempt to call out the name of the other first.

WHAT YOU NEED

A rubber spot marker (optional)
10 – 15 minutes

WHAT TO DO

Separate your gathering into two relatively even groups, and ask each of them to form a circle by holding hands with their partners, facing into the centre. The two circles are not physically linked, but the outside edges of each circle will meet at a designated spot. It is useful to identify this spot – such as a rubber spot marker, the centre circle of a basketball court, or a chalk mark, whatever. Each group just needs to understand that one edge of its circle must pass by this spot at all times.

You then ask each circle to rotate, keeping hold of their partners' hands. It does not matter which direction they travel, but they should travel at an even speed that is comfortable for the least able in the group. From a bird's eye view, it should look as if two circles are spinning and their edges at the closest point are about a metre (3') apart, passing over the designated spot.

At a time of your choosing, call "STOP," or find a way to squeeze into the gap between the two rotating circles, and tap the shoulders of the two people (one from each circle) who are

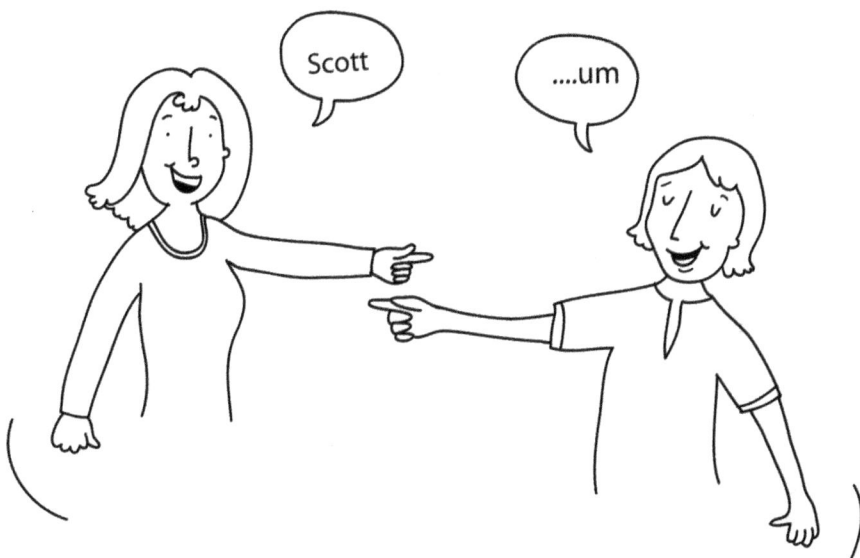

Scott

....um

right now passing over the 'spot.' Everyone else will hear or see this occur, will stop moving, and as quickly as possible, the two tapped people must turn to face one another and try to call the name of the other before they get named. It's fast, high on energy, and you could get dizzy, but it's fun.

From this point, you have at least two options. You could award points to the group when one of its members correctly calls out the name of the other. Or, you could reward this group by 'winning' that other person to join their circle, i.e., your circle gets bigger with every win.

Keep an eye on the speed of the circles. It doesn't take much to whip people around the circle out of excitement, and then you have a real lottery on your hands. Also, if it's too early to ask your group to hold hands, simply let them form a circle and travel in the same direction.

Variations

- Play music, then turn it off (think Musical Chairs) to indicate when the circles have to stop, to identify which two people are closest to the spot.

- Place one circle inside another slightly larger circle, and indicate the spot at which both circles cross. Each circle rotates in a different direction, until you call "STOP."

- As above with two concentric circles – place a hat on one person only (or choose another distinguishing feature) in each circle. On "STOP," the two people with the hats must call out the name of the other person closest to them in the opposite circle. First to call out correctly wins.

WHO IS IT?

If you love a mystery, you'll love this name-game

AT A GLANCE

A group will ask a series of questions that aim to eliminate anyone who does not apply to the answer, to identify the 'mystery' person as quickly as possible.

WHAT YOU NEED

Pen and paper for each person (optional)

5 – 10 mins

WHAT TO DO

This is another one of those contagious 'can-we-do-it-again?' activities. Kids especially love to play this game over and over.

Ask your group to stand any which way in front of you. Explain that you have (in advance) secretly chosen one person in the group to be the 'mystery' candidate. This candidate does not even know that they have been chosen, nor does anyone else. Just you.

Explain that you would now like the group, one at a time, to ask you a question that can only be answered with a "YES" or "NO" reply. If you are not sure of the answer to a question, avoid "Maybe" replies and request that the question be re-phrased. The object for your group is to correctly identify who the mystery person is before, say,

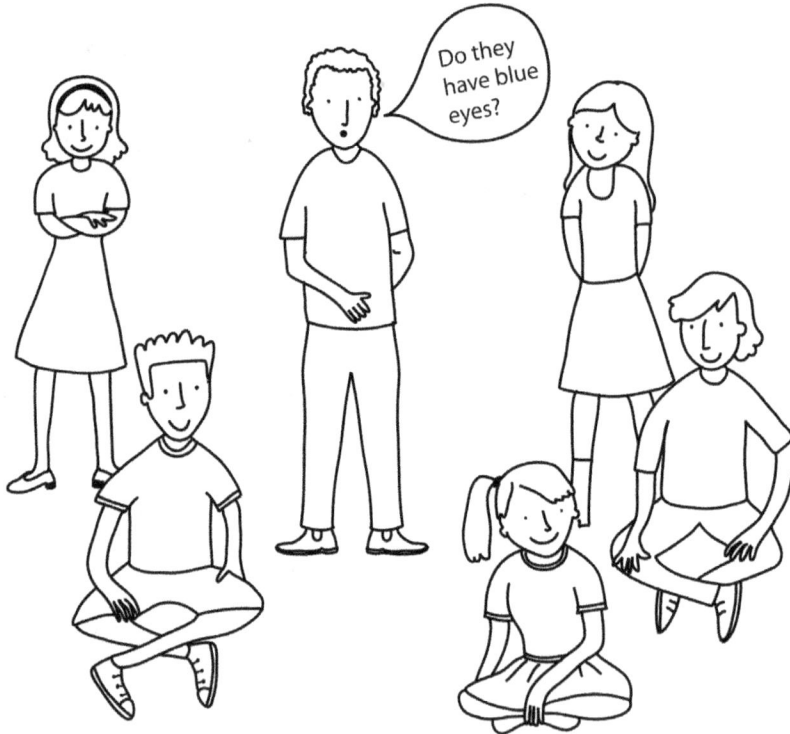

Do they have blue eyes?

ten questions have been asked.

To illustrate, the first question is often gender-related, such as "IS THIS PERSON MALE?" If the person you have chosen is indeed a male, you say "YES," and all of the women in the group sit down. Obviously, if you have chosen a woman, you say "NO" and all the men sit down.

The next question might be, "DO THEY HAVE BLUE EYES?," etc, etc. The questions continue, all aiming to eliminate those who do not fit the description of the mystery person, until one person is left standing and the mystery has been solved.

Anyone can ask a question, even if they are sitting down. After about three or four questions, often less than one-quarter of your group is left standing, so the remaining questions are always probing. Excellent for really getting to know people at a deeper level.

On occasions, one or more individuals will want to make a prediction even though there are stacks of people still standing. Applaud their ingenuity, but ask them instead to construct a question that will result in everyone – other than the person they believe is the mystery person – to sit down.

Variation

In advance, everyone writes their names and an interesting, little known fact about themselves on a piece of paper. You collect and shuffle the papers, and one at a time, read out one of these facts. Game progresses as above.

BUMPITY BUMP BUMP BUMP

One of the funniest name-reminder games I know

AT A GLANCE

Standing in a circle, a person will call out the name of the person to their left or right, or in front of them, or their own name as quickly as possible upon the signal of a person in the middle.

WHAT YOU NEED

5 - 10 mins

WHAT TO DO

Having formed your group into a circle, ask them to repeat after you the words "BUMPITY BUMP BUMP BUMP." I tend to give it a bit of a 'groove' as I say it to impress on my groups that this is very serious stuff – not!

Explain that the person standing in the middle of the circle (in this case, you) will approach anyone in the circle, look them straight in the eye, point to them and exclaim one of the following four words "LEFT," "RIGHT," "YOU" or "ME." Each is an instruction to call out the name of the person to their left or right, their own name, or the name of the person doing the pointing. At this juncture, I typically suggest that everyone should review the names of their neighbours, not to mention mine (the Pointer) and of course their own (the Pointee) – you'll be surprised by how few people actually choose to practice saying their own name; and they won-

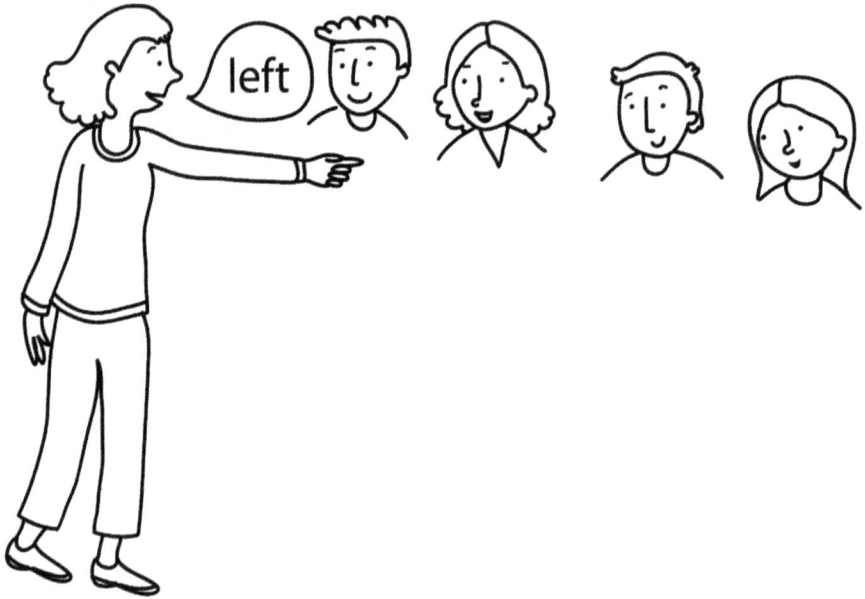

der why they stumble with it later!!

Anyway, to this moment, the game works fine as a name-reminder activity, but it's got no spunk. So this is where the bumps come in. To give the exercise a little edge, the Pointee must attempt to (correctly) name the left-right-you-or-me person as quickly as possible, indeed, before the Pointer can say the words "BUMPITY BUMP BUMP BUMP." So, for example, it could look like this – the Pointer points and calls out, "LEFT," and immediately will follow with "BUMPITY BUMP BUMP BUMP." Meanwhile, the Pointee will attempt to blurt out the name of the person to their left before the Pointer gleefully gets to the final "BUMP."

If the Pointee manages to shout out (note, that most people confuse volume with speed in this activity) the correct name before the last bump, the Pointer hangs his or her head low and moves onto another target. However, if the Pointee is too slow, gives the wrong name, or simply looks like a doe in headlights, everyone has a good laugh, and the Pointer and Pointee swap positions. Once your group 'gets' what's happening, introduce one or more new Pointers into the middle to ramp up the energy and fun.

More than 50 people in your group? Separate into two or more smaller groups, or once you have established the basic naming and bumpity-bump-bump-bump protocols, quickly appoint multiple Pointees to the centre of the circle to generate more activity.

Variations

- For younger groups, or those with lesser name-retention abilities, limit the Pointer to asking for the names of "LEFT" and "RIGHT" neighbours only.
- Add, or substitute the command with "TWO TO YOUR LEFT" or "THREE TO YOUR RIGHT" to really challenge your group.
- Choosing to play for keeps, you could eliminate people as they make mistakes on their journey to the much celebrated name-knowing heaven. Even better, ask those folks who are eliminated to remain in the circle, but to squat down. The game continues as if they were not there, but the gap between people who are still 'in' will cause some of them to overlook who their neighbours truly are, i.e., their next 'left' or 'right' neighbour could be standing half way around the circle.

MOTION NAME-GAME

An oldie-but-still-a-goodie name-game

AT A GLANCE
Standing in a circle, each person in turn will say their name and make a physical movement, after which everyone else will repeat their name and movement.

WHAT YOU NEED
5 – 10 mins

WHAT TO DO
Yeah, yeah, I know, this activity is as old as the hills. Yet, no matter how often I struggle with these thoughts before I reluctantly present it, I am always pleased with the results. Indeed, I have had participants come up to me several years after an event, still remembering my name and my 'motion' at the time. Impressive. You see, our brains think in pictures, not words, so we are far more effective at memory recall when we can associate a picture (of a movement) with new data (a name).

Participants stand in a circle facing each other. One person kicks off (often you) by saying their name loud enough for the group to hear, and then follow it with a physical motion or movement that represents something about that person (you). For example, I will say "MARK" and may follow it with the swing of my arms as if I were holding a tennis racquet to serve a tennis ball.

Upon this introduction, the rest of the group – in unison – will repeat my name while, at the same time, mimicking my movement. Moving clockwise, the person to the left of the newly-introduced will repeat the process, upon which, the group will repeat their name and copy their movement. And so on around the circle.

This is good, but as a further challenge, ask that as each new person is introduced, the group works in reverse and repeats the name and the motion of every known person all the way back to the start. For example, if the fourth

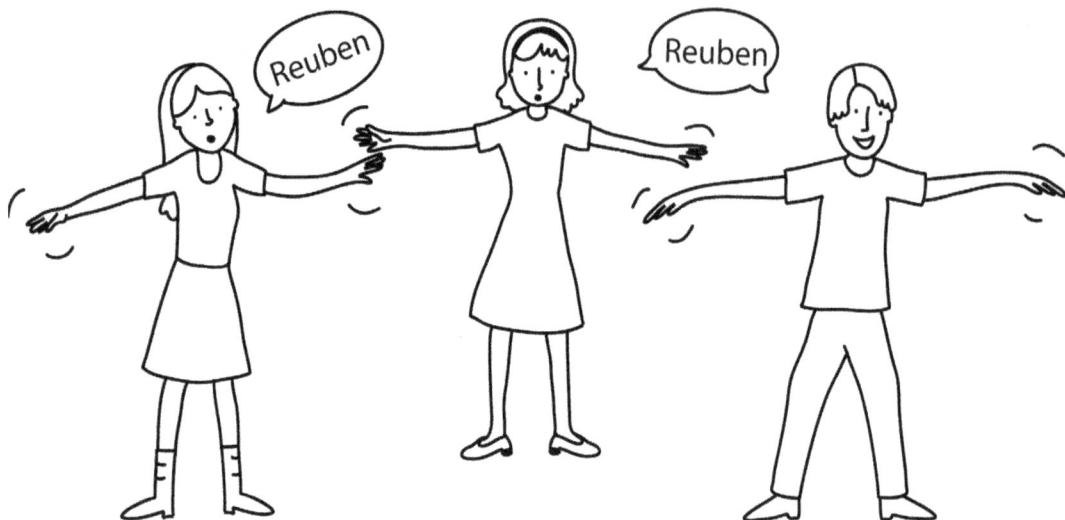

person (Pedro) has just introduced himself, the group may say "PEDRO" (motion), "CHERYL" (motion), "AVRIL" (motion), and finally "MARK" (motion).

I have worked this exercise with up to fifty people in one large circle, and it works a treat. However, this number is rather large, so I suggest that you 'chunk it' with groups of say 20 to 25 people, as described at the start of this section.

Variations

- Add a sound to the motion, e.g., in my case, I will click my tongue as I serve the tennis ball, which of course everyone repeats as they mimic the motion.

- For groups that have a high level of name-knowingness, use middle names and a motion.

- For a deeper connection, invite people to demonstrate a gesture that represents one of their most important values.

- Rather than using a motion, ask each person to introduce themselves by first using an adjective (or favourite fruit / vegetable, value, etc) starting with the initial of their first name, e.g., 'MARVELLOUS MARK" and everyone repeats.

CONCENTRATION

One of those frustrating, yet very fun rhythmic name-games

AT A GLANCE

Sitting in a circle, one person attempts to maintain a certain rhythm or beat as they say their own name twice, and then call the name of another person in the group twice to signal that person's turn.

WHAT YOU NEED

10 – 15 mins

WHAT TO DO

With your group preferably sitting in a circle, establish a beat by asking your group to mimic your movements of SLAP – SLAP (slap open palms on knees) CLICK – CLICK (click own fingers, one at a time, left then right). Practice it a few times, maintaining a constant beat – SLAP – SLAP – CLICK – CLICK – SLAP – SLAP – CLICK – CLICK, and so on.

Next, explain that on the slaps, one person at a time will say their own name twice, that is, they say their own name on each slap. And then, on the clicks, this same person will call out the name of another person sitting in the circle twice, so that with each click the name is called. So, starting with me as an example, it may sound like this "MARK" (slap) "MARK" (slap) "GILL" (left click) "GILL" (right click).

OK, this is where it gets tricky, and will move people to the edge of their seats. The rule is that the person belonging to the name called with the clicks restarts the process immediately. And in the spirit of the game, I do mean immediately – in keeping with the beat. In a perfect world, there will be no surprises, fumbles or stutters as names keep pace.

Continuing the example, Gill will quickly resume with "GILL" (slap) "GILL" (slap) and then call a new person's name with her clicks, such as "TREVOR" (click) "TREVOR" (click). Which is Trevor's cue to wake up, clap and click, etc. Give your group a few mulligan rounds, and then start in earnest. Provided the beat is maintained and names are correctly called, the fun continues. All "errors" earn a hearty round of applause and laughter. The person who erred starts over. Repeat until the level of name-knowingness has peaked.

In the beginning, you will want to keep the pace of the beat rather slow, about two beats per second. As the group warms up, feel free to step on the accelerator.

Apart from struggling with memory loss, often the hardest part of this exercise is to hear the names called out over the din of the slapping and clicking. Remind people to keep their voices loud.

Beyond thirty people, 'chunk it' as de-- scribed at the beginning of this section.

Variation

When someone makes a mistake, this person moves into the seat directly to the left of the person who started (the 'leader'), while everyone between this point and the seat of the person who erred moves up one seat. Everyone aims to progress around the circle to eventually sit in the seat of the 'leader.'

PEEK-A-WHO

A compelling 'name-this-person-quickly name-game

AT A GLANCE
Two people sit facing opposite sides of a large screen held between them, and attempt to name the other person as soon as the screen is pulled to the ground.

WHAT YOU NEED
Large sheet or blanket
10 – 20 mins

WHAT TO DO
Randomly separate your group into two roughly even teams. Got more than 60 people? Designate two or more areas of play, each with about 30 people. After hearing your instructions, each group will operate independently of each other.

Ask for a volunteer to assist you to unfurl a large sheet or blanket (let's call it a screen) in the middle of your playing space, so that it hangs lengthwise and upright with the bottom edge touching the floor. Now, ask each 'team' to sit on one side of the screen, in such a way that no one belonging to the opposing team can be seen. Also, ask anyone sitting close to the screen to scoot back at least two metres (7') from it. This is your basic set-up; you are now ready to play.

Without announcing what is about to happen, invite one person from each group to come forward and sit directly in front of and facing the screen. Explain that on some agreed signal ("3, 2, 1" works fine), the screen will be

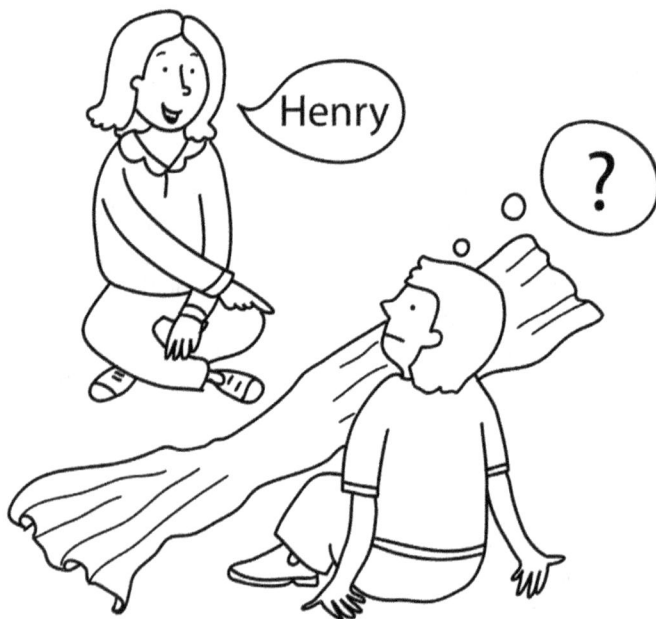

rapidly pulled to the floor between the two rivals, which is their cue to (correctly) name their opponent. Whoever names the other first 'wins' their opponent for their team, i.e., the opponent switches loyalty and joins the winner's team before play resumes.

Invite several individuals to compete for name supremacy, one at a time, and then ramp up the challenge – ask for two people per team to sit facing the screen. This time, the couple who manage to (correctly) name their opponents first (any order, any person) will win.

A word of advice: ensure that one team is not advantaged by a strong backlight which casts a telling silhouette on the screen!

Variations

- Ask one person from each team to sit with their back to the screen, facing their team. This person is not permitted to turn around, but will focus instead on his or her team's efforts to communicate the identity of their opponent using non-verbal 'language' only once the screen has been dropped. In case you're wondering, they can not spell or mouth their opponent's name in any way.

- As above, but this time each team is permitted to speak. Describe anything other than speak the opponent's name.

- The screen remains up at all times. One person from each team will face the screen, and place their right arm under it, so that their opponent can fully see their lower arm. The first to name the other, wins. Oh, and pssst... this is my favourite winning strategy of all time – waiting for the other to proffer a suggestion first, recognise their voice and then respond. A cack!

COCKTAIL PARTY

A quick name reinforcer, and welcome segue to a drinks break

AT A GLANCE

In a limited time frame, people mingle about shaking hands and greeting as many fellow participants by name as possible.

WHAT YOU NEED

1 - 2 mins

WHAT TO DO

Looking for a quick way to wrap up a session, perhaps reinforce a few names people may have just learned, or want to simply cut to a drinks break? This is it.

Invite people to bunch around you, capturing the image of palatial sur-

roundings, evening gowns, black ties and cocktails. Suggest that each person holds in their left hand an imaginary drink, or cocktail if they choose. Then, on your signal, everyone is encouraged to meet, shake the hands of and greet as many people at the party as possible, in say, 43.5 seconds (this is not a magic number!).

On "GO," it will sound something like, "OOOOHH, DARLING, SO GOOD TO SEE YOU!. I'M HAVING A FRIGHTFULLY GOOD TIME......" Chat for a few moments, discuss drinks, recent holidays to the Swiss Alps, and then in typical cocktail party fashion, interrupt the conversation with a "WELL, DORIS, I

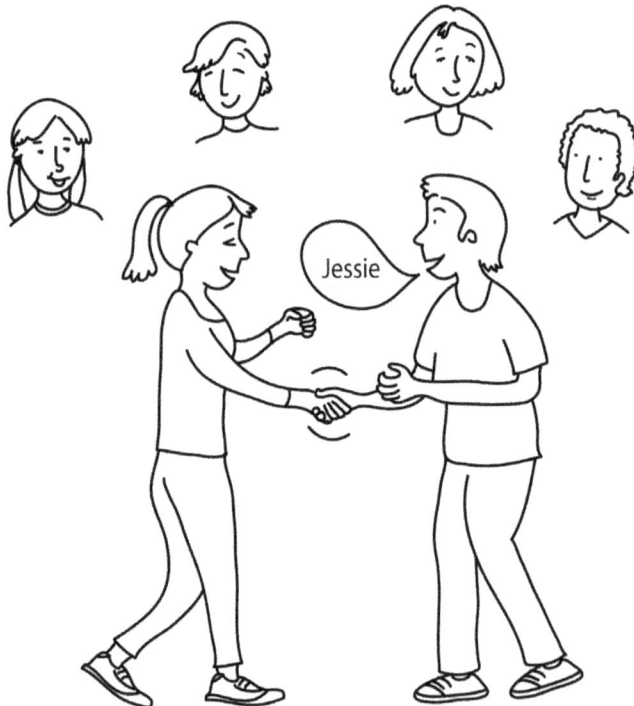

Jessie

MUST KEEP MOVING." Air kiss, kiss (these are not mandatory), and ."..BYE BYE!"...and off you go to greet another party guest.

Suggest to your group that they should use the other person's name as often as possible, enquire about the other person's drink (remember, they are holding on to it), but not spend too long with any one person. For a bit of fun, ask someone for the time and see if they spill their drink!

When you feel like the heat has started to dissipate from the party, quell the action and ask your group what is odd about the activity. Someone will usually remark that "There's nothing in my hand," which is your cue to say...."LET'S REMEDY THAT SITUATION – TIME FOR A DRINKS BREAK."

Variations

- For kids, suggest they are holding their favourite (soft) drink.

- Imagine you are in a swanky Food Hall. Invite people to mingle as they treat themselves to the extraordinary array of fine foods available on people's trays.

INTERACTIVE FUN

You've broken the ice, your group is warmed up, and lots of names are bedded down. Great. You and your group are now ready to have some 'bigger' fun.

The pages that follow comprise a stack of fun, interactive and engaging activities that will involve your whole group at the same time. And, as I often say, if you discover any intrinsic value in these activities beyond the pure, unadulterated pleasure of mixing with a large group of people, let me know!

Activities described in this section typically feature:

- Ample opportunities for group members to interact, play, trust and learn
- Fun and laughter as a major component
- Emphasis on whole group participation / interaction
- Success-oriented activity, not win / lose
- 10 to 30 minutes of play

This section is categorized into three further activity distinctions, in relation to the general nature of the exercise. Within each distinction, a sequence is presented that reflects a gradual increase in the level of interaction, challenge and / or exertion required.

FUNN Interactive Games

Ghost
Alien
Paper Golf
I Pass This Shoe
Genie Game
Chicken-Eyes
Superiority
Instigator
Chocolate Circle
Comet Balls
Evolution
Eliminator
Quick Pass
Finger-Snaps
Jockeys
Have You Ever?
Chic-A-Boom

High Energy Activities

Samurai
The Wave
Everybody's It
Monarch
Octopus Tag
Mad Chefs
Asteroids
Clothes-Peg Tag
Striker
King's Treasure
Water World
Capture the Flags
Ultimate Hand Ball

Team Challenge & Problem-Solving Activities

Circle the Circle
Four Letter Word
Paper Plane Contest
Funny Walk
Dress Me Ups
Pictionary
Leaning Tower of Feetza
Human Machines
Stick Around
Cold Shoulder

GHOST

A perfect quiet-them-down activity that sharpens our hearing and nerves of steel

AT A GLANCE

A small number of people attempt to eliminate others in the group who have their eyes closed by secretly standing behind them for ten seconds without being noticed.

WHAT YOU NEED

10 – 15 mins

WHAT TO DO

During summer camp, I was always looking for activities that would calm the kids down before they went to bed. When things were particularly desperate, I pulled this out this one.

Randomly or otherwise, volunteer a small group of people to be the 'ghosts.' I find one ghost per eight or so people works well. Ask these folks to stand aside for a moment, as you invite the rest of your crew to scatter evenly throughout a specified area. Once positioned, ask everyone (other than the ghosts) to close their eyes. These folks will not be moving anywhere.

Next, you invite the 'ghosts' to enter the area, wandering in and out of the group (with eyes wide open) as quietly as possible. Their goal is to eliminate people from the game. They will do this by standing directly behind one person at a time for ten seconds without being noticed. If ten seconds pass, and they remain unnoticed, the ghost will gently tap the unknowing person on his or her shoulders. At which point, the unknowing normally shrieks and jumps a foot in the air with surprise. The shrieker is now eliminated, and will stand off to the side to enjoy watching others get caught by surprise too. Or not.

It's not as easy at it sounds. Creaking floorboards, shallow breathing, sniffles,

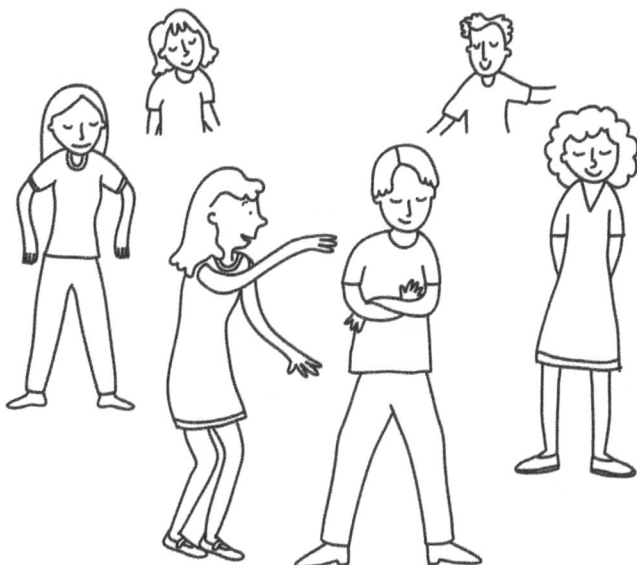

etc have brought undone many a sneaking approach. So, if someone suspects that a ghost is behind them, they may ask "IS THERE A GHOST BEHIND ME?" If they are correct, the ghost and accuser swap roles, i.e., the ghost now closes his or her eyes, and the accuser becomes a ghost. However, if they are wrong, the accuser is eliminated.

Keep going until everyone has been eliminated, or set a time limit for the ghosts to accomplish their task.

Variations

- Limit the accusations of "IS THERE A GHOST BEHIND ME?" to no more than five. This curbs the enthusiasm of those who are lazy and just want to make nearby ghosts wary.
- Separate into pairs, one person with his or her eyes closed, while the other starting about 10 metres (33') away attempts to secretly approach and tap him or her on the shoulder before getting noticed.

ALIEN

A game that can run secretly in the background of any program

AT A GLANCE
A small washer is passed secretly from one person to another in an attempt to not have the item in one's possession when the nominated time expires.

WHAT YOU NEED
One 4 cm (1.5") metal washer

WHAT TO DO
This has got to be one of the simplest, yet most absorbing games I know. Introduce a small metal washer to your group so that everyone gets a good look at it. Then, explain that someone (perhaps you?) will start with the washer in their possession, but will as soon as possible pass it to another person in the group – without their knowing. The idea is to not have the washer in one's possession at a time you declare.

I have introduced the 'alien' washer into highly interactive programs that lasted only two hours, and I have also introduced it into residential camping programs that ran for a week. It works either way.

The key is to hide the washer so that it will be easily found or uncovered. The 'passer' should attempt to place it on another person or their possessions so that the latter will eventually uncover it as part of his or her daily routine. Slipping it into their coat pocket works well, as does placing it inside a lunchbox. I have even seen people slide it into a roll of toilet paper to surprise some random person when they visit the bathroom! However, if the 'passer' notes that the washer has not been detected within a reasonable length of time, they are responsible for retrieving it, and passing it to someplace or someone new.

Note, there is no magic in a washer – you could use any item. But, a washer does have weight, it is relatively flat and thin and it's not the sort of thing you or I generally see lying around – so when it's seen, it is noticeable.

Variations

- To heighten the element of secrecy, alert your group to the fact that if someone is caught in the act of passing the washer, the 'passer' must pass the washer to another person.

- Use two or more washers simultaneously. I sometimes do this without notice to ramp up the fun!

PAPER GOLF

A form of golf that everyone can play

AT A GLANCE
Having designed their own personal three-hole golf course on paper, each person invites one or more people to play a round using a pen to mark the progress of their golf balls.

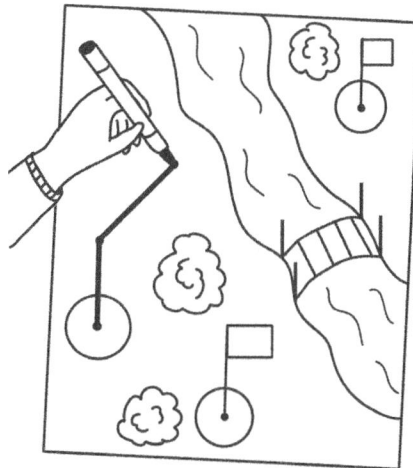

WHAT YOU NEED
Sheet of paper for each person
Markers or pens to share
20 – 30 mins

WHAT TO DO
This exercise starts with people on their own, moves them into pairs, and can then build to three or more people.

Hand out a sheet of paper, the larger the better, for each person. Then, using paper in front of you to demonstrate, explain that you would like everyone to design their own golf course. For those who, like me, don't really play golf, describe all the common features of a typical golf course as you draw them on your paper.

I suggest designing a golf course with just three holes, but there's no magic in this number. Just be sure to add tees, fairways, greens and holes with little flags poking out of them. Design a few challenging hazards such as lakes, streams, and sand bunkers, in addition to local flora and fauna such as gum trees and a roaming kangaroo. Other than those seriously creative types, five or so minutes is sufficient time for most people to design their very own championship standard (paper) golf course.

Now, to play. With pen or marker in hand, starting with the tip of the pen on the first tee, players close their eyes, and move the pen across the paper (so that it marks a line), stopping whenever it seems necessary (such as to avoid a water hole, or running off the paper). Players open their eyes, and record this as their first stroke. Upon reassessing the terrain, players place their pen at the very end of the last 'stroke,' close their eyes and take another shot. Although each golf course designer may implement their own rules, the general idea is to avoid hitting or crossing their pen over any of the drawn obstacles.

Play continues until the end of a single stroke (line) lands directly in the middle of the first hole. Crossing over or skimming the edge of the hole doesn't count, the pen must land right in it. Oh, and golf balls do swing, so reasonable curves are okay – 90 degree angles are not.

Ordinarily, golfing partners will take turns at swinging. When the Club House is finally reached, add the total number of swings (lines) taken, and the player with the lowest score wins.

Groups of up to four or five people can play on a single paper golf course.

Variation

Rather than leading the pen across the paper course, a player will use one finger to hold the pen upright and push it forward so that the tip slides across the paper leaving a diminishing trail of ink. This method will require many more 'swings,' and some compromise on exactly where the end of the 'stroke' is.

I PASS THIS SHOE

A ridiculously fun way to fill in a few minutes

AT A GLANCE
Sitting in a circle on the floor, people pass a shoe from their right to their left to a particular beat while singing a little ditty.

WHAT YOU NEED
A shoe for each person
10 – 15 mins

WHAT TO DO
Form a circle, and invite everyone to sit on the floor, and then ask them to take off one of their shoes and place it on the floor directly in front of them. At this point, I explain that I would like to teach everyone to sing a little ditty

with me. It's very simple, it goes something like this:

"I PASS THIS SHOE FROM ME TO YOU. I PASS LIKE THIS AND I NEVER, NEVER MISS."

Imagine me singing this tune, swinging my head slightly to the left and right as if keeping time to a beat. Basically, there's one beat for every word, except for the words "AND I" in the second line which is treated as one beat together. Practice singing this a few times, and then introduce the shoes for the first time, asking everyone to copy what you are about to show them.

Clearly demonstrating, I hold my own shoe in front of me, and starting with an elongated "IIIIII..." (to signal the start of the song), I physically pass my shoe to my left hand neighbour. And then on "PASS" (the second word of the tune), I place this shoe in front of them. On "THIS" I pick up the shoe that now sits in front of me (with thanks to my right-hand neighbour), and pass it to my left hand neighbour, and so on, for the whole song. Basically, you pick up or pass a shoe for every beat of the song. Err, except on one occasion!

Do practice the full stanza at least once before you get to the fun part. Then, announce the dead-beat 'Never-Nevers' as I like to call them. Explain that when your group has picked up the shoe in front of them on the "AND-I" beat in the second line of the tune (just before "NEVER, NEVER"), they must hold onto the shoe for two full beats. So, they will pick up the shoe on "AND I," tap the shoe in front of their left neighbour on "NEVER." Still holding the same shoe, they tap it in front of themselves on the second "NEVER," and finally pass and place the shoe in front of their neighbour on "MISS." You will definitely need to practice this little 'hiccup' in procedures.

The whole point of this exercise is to sing five full stanzas of the tune while passing the shoes correctly. Yeah, right! As you might imagine, it rarely happens, as people often get tripped up on the "Never-Nevers."

Thanks to Jim Schoel for passing this old shoe to me!

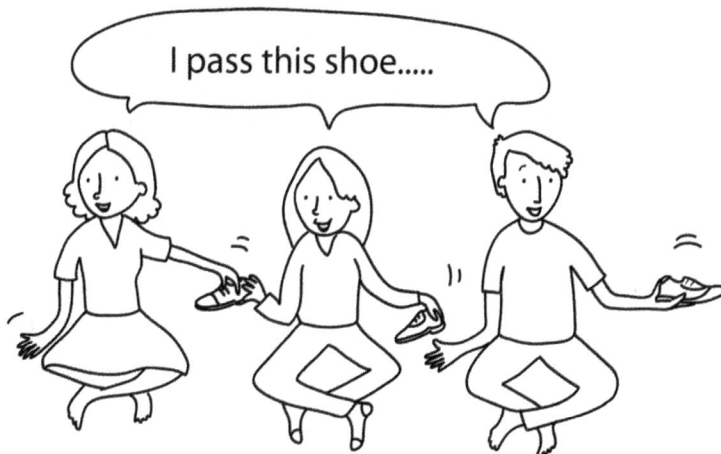

I pass this shoe.....

Variations

- Got no shoes? Then, distribute an array of different-sized soft objects. Much like shoes, passing a variety of shapes, weights and sizes is ideal for testing your group's passing prowess.

- Two shoes in front of each person, using two hands, one shoe goes one direction, the other the opposite direction. Arghhhh....

GENIE GAME

A perfect 'something' to fill-in two minutes

AT A GLANCE

Standing in a circle, three people will quickly react to the signal of the present 'Genie' to shape their bodies as if they were 'striking a gong,' before passing the signal onto another three people in the group.

WHAT YOU NEED

2 – 10 mins

WHAT TO DO

Start by forming a circle in which everyone can clearly see every other person. Beyond 40 people, this can be tricky, so I suggest separating into two or more smaller groups after you have briefed the activity. Works best if your group is standing, but sitting can be okay (just ask all those involved in movements to stand as they do them).

You kick off by placing your arms high in the air above your head, elbows bent and the palms of your hands pressed against each other. You could then move your head to the left and right and look like a Genie, in fact you should – it's fun, and all part of the game.

Now, explain that as a Genie, you have the power to cast a spell on anyone else in the group so that they immediately become a Genie too. You do this by simply lowering your hands (still pressed together), and pointing them towards any other person in the group. This person will immediately mimic your look, and raise arms above head, and rock his or her head from side to side Genie-like too. At this point, the 'old' Genie (you) can resume a normal standing-in-a-circle position.

As soon as a new Genie is identified, his or her two neighbours must immediately assume the 'clanging gong' position (as I like to call it), which

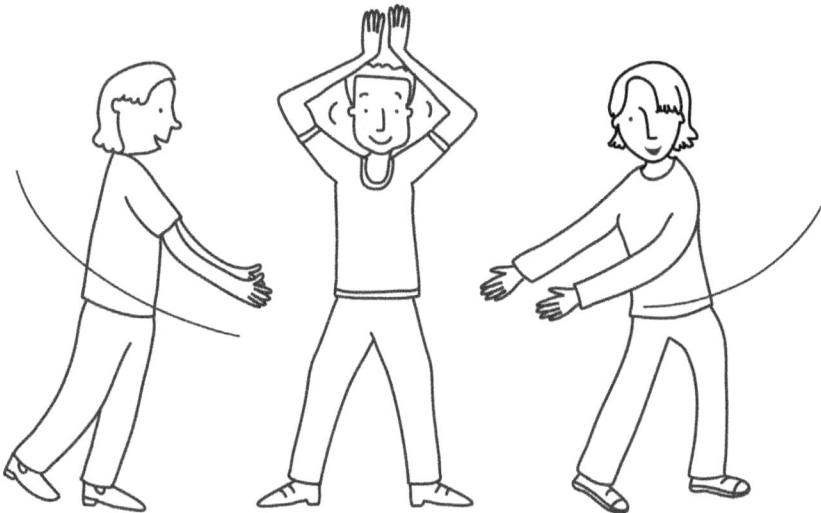

involves each person swinging their two arms towards the Genie as if they were banging a gong resting on his or her tummy. They don't actually touch the Genie – but thanks for asking.

Then, quick as a flash, the Genie points to a new person in the circle, and the process repeats itself over and over again. The key is to maintain a consistent rhythm of pointing and clanging, the quicker the better.

You'll probably squeeze a good two or so minutes out of this silliness, which is all it is. Its raison d'être is observed simply in the hilarity generated when someone makes a mistake. There's no more serious consequence than a good laugh.

Variation

Same deal, but introduce eliminations for a slow or inaccurate Genie or clanging movements. Rather than removing people from the group as they are eliminated, ask the error-inclined people to fold their arms on their chests to present a further challenge for those still in the game to identify their true 'neighbours.'

CHICKEN-EYES

Another great excuse for filling in some down-time

AT A GLANCE
Standing in a circle, an impulse of kooky 'chicken-eye' actions are passed as quickly as possible from one person to another in a particular direction, until the direction is reversed or some-one makes an error.

WHAT YOU NEED
2 – 5 mins

WHAT TO DO
To start, ask your group to practice what I call 'chicken-eyes,' where you make a circle with your index finger and thumb (on both hands), splaying all other fingers, and then placing the circles over your eyes. Check it out, you should be looking at a group of chickens all wearing gorgeous horn-rimmed glasses!

Form a circle – standing close to one another works best – and announce that you will initiate the first set of chicken-eyes. You pull just one hand up, form one chicken-eye and place it over the corresponding eye. That is, if I use my right hand to form the eye, I place it over my right eye. Next, explain that as a result of using my right hand, this will dictate the direction of the chicken-eye impulse. So, the neighbour to my right will now continue the action and perform a chicken-eye too. And so on it goes.

This is all cool, except heading in one direction all the time will soon get boring. So explain that the impulse of chicken-eyes may at any time be passed in one of three ways to elicit a particular response:

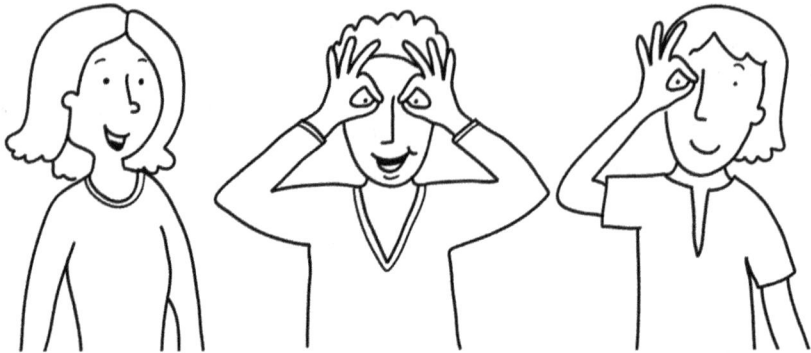

- To continue the impulse in the same direction – place chicken-eye over the corresponding eye;
- To reverse the direction – use other arm / hand to place chicken-eye over other eye, i.e., if direction was running to the right, use left hand over left eye to reverse direction; and
- To skip the next person (i.e., their neighbour) continuing in the same direction – use both hands to form two eyes.

The key is to respond to the impulse as quickly as possible, sending the impulse of a chicken-eye or eyes around the circle at break-neck speed. The most fun is allowing the action to swing this way and that for as long as you've got people's attention. When an error occurs – such as responding too slowly, or responding when they shouldn't – the person to the left of where the error occurred may resume the action.

Got a really large group? No trouble, just initiate several 'chicken-eyes' simultaneously. What happens when two impulses meet? Craziness and a lot of laughter. Perfect.

Variations

- Instruct people to call out "B'GAWK" (you know, the sound of a chicken) as they perform a chicken-eye.
- Rather than eliminating people who make an error, invite them to run around the outside of the circle flapping their arms as if they were chickens and either (a) return to their spot once they have completed one rotation and then rejoin the action, or (b) keep running until someone else makes a mistake. Either way, the impulse resumes as soon as this person leaves the circle.

SUPERIORITY

A brain-numbing 'I-do-this-you-do-that' activity

AT A GLANCE

Standing in a circle, an individual will attempt to respond quickly with the appropriate 'superior' action to one of three actions performed by an 'Initiator,' lest they be eliminated.

WHAT YOU NEED

10 – 15 mins

WHAT TO DO

I could just tell my group what to do, but it's much more fun to tell a story – that is, a story that I've just made up that features three levels of 'superiority.' I'll share my favourite in a moment, but you can invent any story that appears to make sense and can accommodate a series of fun physical gestures.

I love to tell the story of the fox and how it is considered sacred in China. To anchor the fox in the story, I will invite my group to mimic my actions, of holding my slightly-cupped hands atop of my head to depict fox ears. Next, I explain that the only thing superior to the fox is a fox-trap, and will extend both of my arms out in front of me, one of top of the other, opening and closing as if they were the jaws of a very large trap. Again, I ask everyone to mimic my actions. Continuing the story, I suggest that 'human beings' are superior to traps because we know to avoid them. For 'humans,' I stand upright and quickly place my hands on my upper thighs. Finally, the only thing superior to a human being is the fox, because it is sacred in China. Get it? Much like Ro-Sham-Bo (see page 95), one thing is always superior to another.

OK. Assemble your group into a circle, and invite one person to start in the middle. This middle person (the 'Initiator') will directly approach someone standing in the circle and will quickly demonstrate one of the three levels of superiority – the fox, the trap or the human. Immediately, upon seeing this action, the person they approach (the 'Responder') must demonstrate the superior action. For example, if the Initiator showed a fox, the Responder would have to rapidly show the trap.

As your group starts to grasp the concept, you can be assured of plenty of laughs. Basically, if the Responder is slow or demonstrates the wrong action, they are invited to have some fun in the centre and swap with the Initiator. After a few minutes, ramp up the action by introducing two, three or more Initiators.

As with many form-a-circle activities, if you have a really large group, describe the activity, split 'em up and allow each small group to play independently. For interaction purposes, swap one half of a group into another group several times.

Variations

- Styled as an elimination, if the Responder acts too slowly or incorrectly, they are asked to leave the circle and watch the action continue until a 'showdown' occurs between the final two people.

- Allow your group to mix and mingle. Two people approach one another, decide who will be the Initiator and then act accordingly. Suggest that people alternate roles, so that if they have just been a Responder, they get to be the Initiator when they next meet a partner.

INSTIGATOR

An active 'follow-the-leader' exercise that sharpens observation skills

AT A GLANCE

A person watches a group of people mingling with one another, yet moving in exactly the same manner, and attempts to guess which one person is leading the series of changes in the group's movements.

WHAT YOU NEED

10 – 15 mins

WHAT TO DO

Play this just for kicks, or if you particularly want to develop and sharpen your group's focus and observation skills. Form a circle and explain that one person will soon be designated as the 'Instigator' whose role is to initiate a series of movements which the rest of the group will copy. It is critical that the others follow the Instigator's movements exactly, and adopt any changes as soon as they become aware of them.

The trick is that the identity of the Instigator needs to remain secret, because a second person who will volunteer to be the first 'Bunny' will not know who the Instigator is. Once nominated, the Bunny will either leave the room, turn around, or close his or her eyes while the group nominates who will be their Instigator, i.e., this can be done silently by simply pointing at someone.

To start, invite your group to mingle among themselves within a defined area. Just prior to the Bunny entering this realm, the Instigator will begin a series of movements, such as flapping his or her arms, poking out the tongue or walking in a particular way. Then, the Bunny will enter and, from a safe distance, simply look at everyone and their movements. The group will continue to mingle and maintain the current movement at all times, while secretly stealing a glance at the Instigator (or other early-adopter) from time to time to pick up any changes in the movement. The Instigator should try to change his or her movements every ten seconds or so. Big moves are best and the most fun to watch.

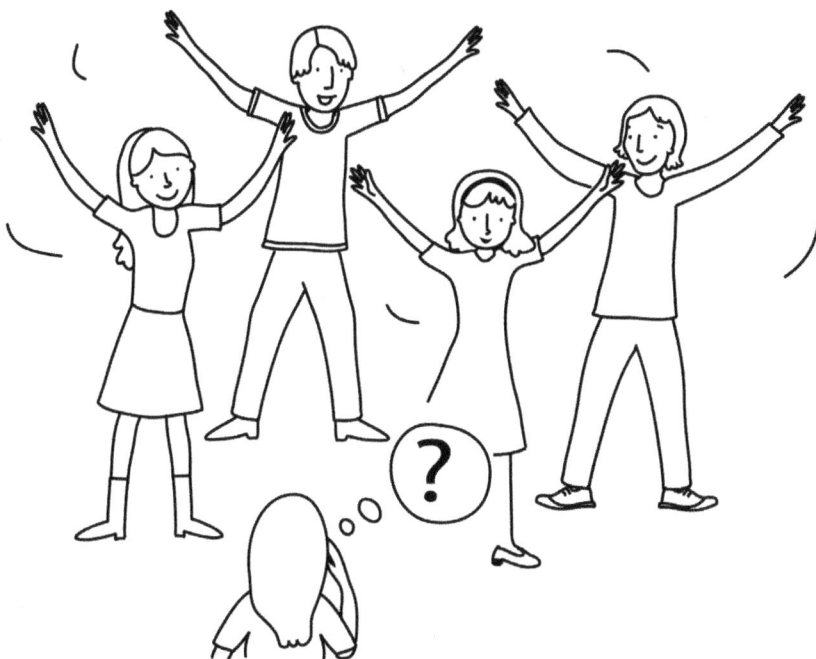

Naturally, your group must be careful not to make their glances at the Instigator too obvious too early. Give the Bunny four 'official' guesses, and once the Instigator is correctly identified, ask for a new person to volunteer to be the next Bunny. Play several rounds.

Variations

- Invite the Instigator to become the Bunny after he or she has been discovered.

- If you have a high-performance group, ask the Instigator to be a 'statue' moving from one frozen position to another. A hint – best time to move is when the Bunny isn't looking.

CHOCOLATE CIRCLE

A crazy dice game that will suit every sweet tooth in your group

AT A GLANCE

Sitting in a circle, people take turns rolling a dice. If an individual rolls a 6, he or she will attempt to eat the chocolate before someone else rolls a 6.

WHAT YOU NEED

One dice

Several items of clothing, e.g., hat, t-shirt, scarf, etc

Knife and fork

Block of chocolate

Tray

15 – 30 mins

WHAT TO DO

The clothing I refer to here should be relatively easy to put on and take off, that's why I suggest a hat, scarf, and a t-shirt. Sun-glasses, a coat, and gloves are also good possibilities.

Ask your group to sit in a circle – on the floor / ground works best. Place a tray in the middle of the circle, with the knife, fork and block of chocolate

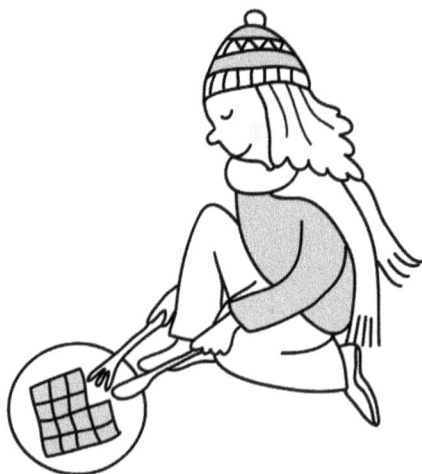

sitting atop. Adjacent to the tray, place the clothing.

Explain that one at a time, each person will roll the dice, and regardless of the result, the dice will be passed to the left around the circle. Nothing happens unless someone rolls a 6, at which point (after passing the dice), the lucky roller gets up and races into the centre of the circle. They are now 'entitled' to eat the chocolate, but, they must put on all of the clothing first, and then only touch the chocolate with the knife and fork. That is, fully clothed, the lucky person will attempt to eat one square of chocolate cut from the block using only the knife and fork supplied. It's not as easy as it seems.

This lucky person may continue to eat one square of chocolate at a time, for as long as no one else in the circle rolls a 6. As soon as this event occurs, the person already in the centre must immediately stop doing whatever he or she was doing, and return to their spot in the circle, making room for the new lucky person.

It is highly likely that a 'lucky' person may only get as far as throwing the scarf on before the next 6 is rolled. Then, of course, I have also seen many squares of chocolate consumed by one person in what seemed like a drought of sixes.

Continue until the chocolate disappears or the energy wanes.

With a really large group, introduce two or more dice into the circle (roughly one for every 15 to 20 people) to keep as many people engaged as possible.

Variation

As above, but also wrap the block of chocolate as many times as possible with newspaper or other wrapping paper (to slow the process), as you would with 'Pass the Parcel.' As an added effect, don't tell your group what is wrapped inside.

COMET BALLS

Ideal as an 'arrival activity' while you wait for the later-comers

AT A GLANCE
Individuals toss a knee-high nylon stocking filled with a tennis ball high into the air, aiming to catch it by the tail on its descent.

WHAT YOU NEED
A knee-high nylon stocking, filled with an old tennis ball for each person
15 to 30 mins

WHAT TO DO
Now, I'm not saying you should raid your mother's wardrobe, but you do need stockings for this activity – lots of them – the knee-high kind, and preferably the neon-colour style. The flesh-coloured ones do work; they're just not as exciting.

Fill the toe-end of each stocking with an old tennis ball, and swing it around a few times to really push that sucker to the end. Multiply this effort by as many people in your group, and you are ready to go.

Asking your group to back up a little, demonstrate the unique comet ball swing, by holding the 'tail' of the comet (open end of stocking) in one hand, and then twirling the ball centrifugally around your hand perpendicular to the ground. Huh? Look at the illustration.

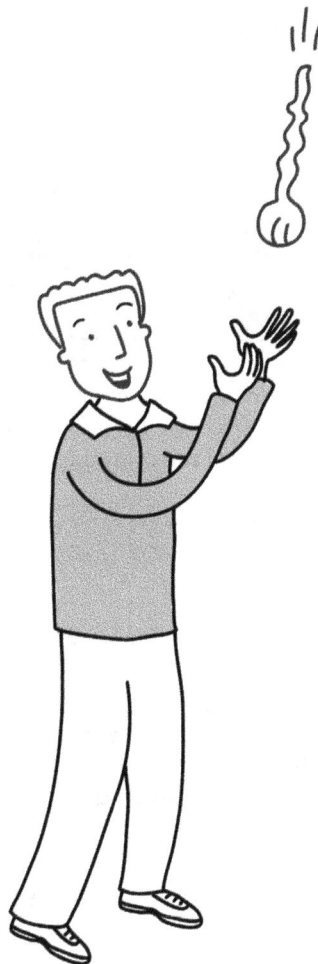

Now, this is the tricky part. Your goal is to time your release so that the comet launches into the air, and does not sail squarely into the ground, or worse, into your group! If successful, you will notice that as it flies, it does look a bit like a comet soaring through the night sky, i.e., ball of fire with a flapping tail. Ultimately, you want to catch the comet by its tail just milliseconds before it hits the ground.

OK. Time to turn it over to your group. Start with one comet per person, and challenge them to catch their own comet. Then, invite two people to join and simultaneously toss and catch their partner's comet.

Ideal as an activity in its own right, or as an 'arrival' activity to occupy and reward those folks who turn up on time. Either way, you will quickly discover how contagious comets are!

Two thoughts. Speak to your local tennis club and ask if you could have their old tennis balls for free, as they are often thrown away! Also, go directly to a stocking manufacturer and ask for a bulk discount; again, they are often quite obliging.

Variations

- Team Comet Ball: Separate your group into two groups, and supply only one 'team' with comets. Separate each team about 30 metres (100') apart from the other. On an agreed signal, all of the comets are launched, and the other team aims to catch as many as possible. Keep score. Repeat several times.

- Comet Horseshoes: Place a hula-hoop (or other receptacle) at two ends of your playing space, about 20 metres (65') apart. Armed with a bunch of comets, divide your group into two, with each half standing behind one of the hoops. Each 'team' aims to bounce as many comets (not just the tail) inside the opposing hoop (the one furthest away) in 5 to 10 minutes.

EVOLUTION

One of my all-time favourite FUNN activities

AT A GLANCE

Physically portraying one of five distinct evolutionary creatures, a person attempts to win a quick game of 'rock-paper-scissors' with other like creatures, to elevate their status and ultimately become a 'supreme' being.

WHAT YOU NEED

10 – 15 mins

WHAT TO DO

Feel free to spin whatever story you choose to introduce this game, the wilder the better. Here's my take on the evolutionary cycle.

Ask your group to help you create five evolutionary creatures. At the bottom of the food chain, we have the egg, followed by the chicken, then the dinosaur, then a Ninja Turtle (the ultimate human being!), and finally, the all-knowing Supreme Being.

Each of these creatures has a unique physical representation. Invite your group to copy these movements and sounds as you show them. It's way fun, and besides, you look funny doing them on your own.

Egg – crouch down into a little ball with legs, and make muffled "EEK-EEK" sounds.

Chicken – flap your arms by your sides and make clucking sounds.

Dinosaur – raise your arms above your head, take big heavy strides and make scary noises.

Ninja Turtle – make like a kung-fu champion slicing the air with lots of karate chops and kicks.

Supreme Being – fold your arms like a genie, look calm and wise.

Now, explain that everyone will start the evolutionary cycle at the lowest level – the egg. To progress through the five phases, each creature must find another like-creature (not too hard in the beginning), and play a quick round of 'rock-paper-scissors.' Whoever wins the round, steps up one evolutionary phase, and the 'loser' will step down a phase. In the case of an egg, there is no lower phase, so if an egg loses a round, they just stay as an egg.

Everyone wants to become a Supreme Being, i.e., to do this, two ninja turtles must face off, and play a game of 'rock-paper-scissors' – the winner becomes Supreme, and the loser returns to being a dinosaur.

Once you become Supreme, you are no longer required to play (Supreme Beings are above this nonsense), and they can simply stand out to the side with their arms crossed looking very self-righteous. Note, it's not possible to have everyone achieve Supreme Being status (nor is this desirable!), so plan to wrap the game up when you sense most people have had enough.

Variation

For a more continuous format, invite Supreme Beings to match wits with one another, i.e., play a game of 'rock-paper-scissors,' and the winner remains supreme, but the loser goes back to being an egg!

ELIMINATOR

The classic game of 'cloak and dagger' where no-one gets hurt

AT A GLANCE

One person, who has been secretly appointed as 'It,' attempts to eliminate everyone in the group – before their identity is revealed – by employing a subtle gesture as they mingle with the group.

WHAT YOU NEED

Deck of playing cards (optional)
5 to 30 mins

WHAT TO DO

I know I say this a lot, but I love this game. And so do large groups.

Upon seizing your group's attention, explain that, in a few moments, some-one in this very room / playing field / space will start eliminating people, one by one. And this 'assassin,' 'It' person or other politically correct term you choose to use, will do this by simply winking at them. Do a quick demonstration to indicate what it looks like.

After secretly appointing your 'It,' invite everyone (including the 'It') to simply mingle about an area, in and out, in and out, politely looking and nodding at others as they pass them by. At some point, the 'It' person will strike and wink at some poor unsuspecting soul. Explain that, to allow time for the 'It' to move away from the scene of the crime, the victim must wait at least five seconds upon receiving the wink, and then exhale a blood-curdling scream, buckle at the knees and collapse on the floor where they stood. Naturally, the more histrionic the 'death' the better.

Meanwhile, the 'It' goes on his or her merry way, aiming to eliminate everyone before his or her identity is revealed (perhaps with some sloppy winking, or clever sleuthing). The general populace, on the other hand, wants to catch the culprit as soon as possible, and they do this by way of accusations. At any time, anyone who is still alive (obviously) may stop their mingling, raise their hand up high and shout "I ACCUSE." At this point, you (the leader) will immediately ask everyone to pause, and ask "IS THERE A SECONDER?" to procure another living mortal to join in the accusation. One of two things will occur:

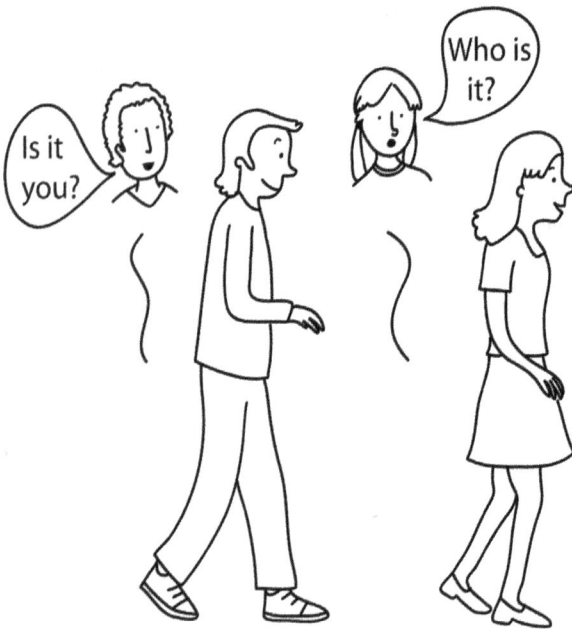

1. No one seconds the accusation. Hence, the accusation cannot be made, everyone returns to their mingling, and it is highly possible the 'it' may now try to eliminate the accuser; or

2. A second person raises their hand to support the accusation. At which point, the leader calls "1, 2, 3" and both accusers must immediately lower their arms (simultaneously) to point directly to the person they believe is the 'It.' If they both point to the same person and he or she is 'It,' the game is over. However, if the two accusers point at different people (even if one of them is pointing at 'It'), they are both eliminated. Uh-oh.

Clearly, a heavy penalty for making an accusation is levied to prevent scurrilous allegations.

Play several rounds, and if you have time, introduce a new weapon of choice (see variations).

So, how do you secretly appoint your 'It' person? Shuffle a deck of cards, hand them out face down and whoever picks a particular card (say, the Ace of Spades) is 'It.' Or, for a no-props style appointment, ask your group to bunch in really close and place their upright thumbs into the centre of a tight throng. Everyone closes their eyes (or turns away from the middle), and you pass your hand over the area and pick a random thumb to squeeze once. The person belonging to this thumb then passes his or her hand over the throng seeking a second random thumb (remember, no one can see this happening), and squeezes it twice. Ta da! The person who belongs to the twice-squoozed thumb is 'It.'

A few quick points. The 'It' person does not have to act on their instinct all the time – indeed, they should not. And, someone who has just been 'hit,' while not technically 'dead' yet (at least in the eyes of the public), can not make an accusation.

Variations

- Introduce the 'Kiss of Death.' The 'It' person puckers their lips as if he or she was blowing a kiss to their victim. Just hilarious, especially watching the 'It' person after you have been eliminated.

- Introduce the 'deadly handshake.' 'It' affects their prey by pressing their index finger against the inside of their victim's wrist several times as they shake hands. It's really creepy. Naturally, in this version, everyone will shake hands many, many times as they mingle in the group.

- Introduce a simple hand gesture, that when observed by others will eliminate them. For example, if the 'It' person places the upside-down 'OK' hand-gesture (using their thumb and fingers of one hand) anywhere below their waist, any unsuspecting person who looks directly at the gesture will be eliminated.

- Multi-day Eliminator. That's right, give the 'It' two or more days to eliminate the group. Choose your preferred style of hit. Allow victims to take their time and plan a really creative, public 'death.' Perfect for residential programs.

QUICK PASS

A fantastic activity to sharpen reflexes and boost people's energy

AT A GLANCE

Sitting in a circle, people pass a variety of items in both directions as quickly as they can, aiming to not end up with two or more items in their lap at the same time.

WHAT YOU NEED

A bag of soft tossable items
5 – 10 mins

WHAT TO DO

Looking to fill a few minutes? Perhaps your group's energy is starting to flag? Try this one on for size.

Sitting in a circle works best for this exercise because you need an obvious place to rest the bevy of items that are about to be liberated.

Distribute one soft tossable item for every three or four people you have in your group. Ask everyone to take a seat, if not already seated, and explain that on "GO" you want all of the people holding an item to 'pass' it to one of their two neighbours.

Now, good passing protocol suggests that a successful pass is one that is placed gently onto the lap of a neighbour (not slammed), perhaps even dropped. If necessary, to avoid issues of inappropriate touching (even if not intended), suggest a mandatory dropping of items onto laps instead. The direction does not matter. Indeed, an item can be passed in any direction by any person at any time.

The goal for each person is to avoid having more than one item in their possession (including their lap) at any point in time. However, to ramp up the fun, when this event does occur for someone, they are obliged to emit a little 'shriek' of some kind to alert others to their plight.

Add more items to increase the challenge, or eliminate people who emit the obligatory "EEEK" to make the circle progressively smaller.

Variations

- If someone is caught, their penalty is to stand up and sit down quickly every time they pass all future items. If it happens again, add a rapid 360 degree turn to the first penalty.

- Limit the number of tossables to one per six to eight people. Instruct that all items must travel in the same direction, with each object aiming to chase down and touch the one ahead of it.

FINGER-SNAPS

A contagious medley of activities that offers massive value for money

AT A GLANCE

A series of fun, interactive activities using small pieces of foam noodles that begin simply and become progressively more 'team' oriented

WHAT YOU NEED

One or two foam noodles

20 – 40 mins

WHAT TO DO

When I first saw this prop introduced, it was like being a five-year old boy all over again. I love this game, and so has every group I've had the pleasure to present it to.

You know those long, bendy foam 'noodles' you see hanging around swimming pools? Grab a couple. I have found that the noodles with a small hole that runs the length of the noodle work best, but it's not a biggie. Take a serrated knife and laying the noodle long ways in front of you, slice it into 25 mm (1") pieces.

Then, lay each piece cut-side down, and cut the circle in half to provide two semi-circle 'finger-snaps' as my friend Ryan McCormack calls them. Why? Because when you hold the semi-circle (curved side facing up) between your thumb and index finger, and squeeze, they SNAP out of your fingers. It's so cool. And this should be your first port of entry to introduce your group into this exercise.

After a minute or so of snapping all over the place, present one or more of the following sequences of awesome 'finger-snapping' activities:

- Join with a partner, and launch and catch one another's finger-snaps simultaneously.

- One pair joins with another pair, to make a finger-snapping quad.

- A quad joins with a quad, to make a finger-snapping octuplet, attempting to snap and catch as many of their group's finger-snaps as possible.

- Bunch everyone into the centre, armed with at least one finger snap each. On "GO," everyone aims to score a point by popping their finger-snap into the back of another person. When a player scores ten points, they are entitled to run around the area with their arms flailing in the air shouting "I'VE GOT TEN, I'VE GOT TEN" over and over.

- Adding to above, all those who have scored ten points, now aim to score another ten points but only by popping their finger-snap into the back of another "I'VE-GOT-TEN" colleague.

- Form pairs, with each partnership holding six to eight finger-snaps each. The goal is to construct a "foam bridge" of four to six snaps – laid side-to-side – held gently between one out-stretched index finger of each person. It's precarious, and it's meant to be. Next, invite each pair to move around the area, aiming to move their bridge in all directions without the bridge collapsing. Now to the fun part!

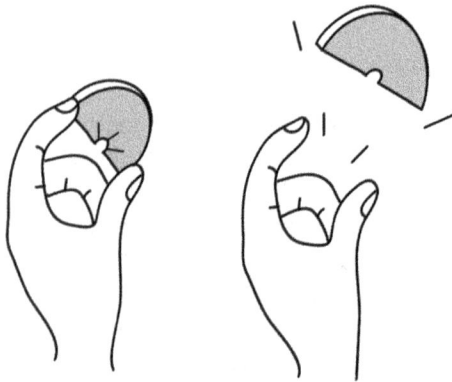

them. A pair can only pop a finger-snap if their bridge is intact.

- Don't have enough finger-snaps to go around? Set up as described above, but this time, any person supporting an intact foam bridge may use their outstretched index finger to hit another pair's bridge. No defending or hovering of bridges is allowed. The only defence is to move the bridge safely out of the way.

Armed with a finger-snap in their outside unoccupied hands, invite each pair to pop this finger-snap at one or more bridges belonging to other people with an aim to 'bust'

Phew! And this is just the beginning. This prop is still new to me, so there has to be a ton of new finger-snapping ideas just waiting to be discovered. And when you do discover them, please tell me!

Variation

You still want more? OK, form a circle, a finger-snap prepared for launch in each hand, and on "GO," create a cacophony of snaps as the impulse travels around the circle. If you close your eyes, it can sound like popcorn or fireworks.

JOCKEYS

Fast-paced action game that never fails to raise a sweat or a smile

AT A GLANCE

On a given signal, two people working as partners will assume one of three physical poses as quickly as possible to avoid being eliminated.

WHAT YOU NEED

15 – 20 mins

WHAT TO DO

Given the fast-paced action that this exercise requires, sequence it appro-

priately and consider the physical attributes of your group before charging forward.

Working in pairs, ask your group to form a large circle where one person stands facing into the circle, and their partner stands directly behind them. You should end up with two circles, one inside the other.

Explain that the person standing behind their partner is the 'Jockey,' while the other is the 'Horse' – for now! Furthermore, as with all racing, you are looking for the fastest horse and jockey combination, and to achieve this goal, you will call one of a series of commands. To prepare for the race, describe these three commands:

- "JOCKEYS UP": the Jockey will jump onto the back of the Horse
- "JOCKEYS DOWN": the Jockey dismounts the Horse
- "SWITCH": the Jockey and Horse switch positions (and therefore immediate roles).

The fourth (and final) command is "RACING," which will oblige the Jockeys to run around the outside of the circle (the Horses) as quickly as they can and resume their standing-behind-their Horse position. Their aim is to not be the last person to return to their 'stable,' lest they eliminated. Once eliminated, the unfulfilled horse or jockey is entitled to give the next series of calls.

To be clear, if the Jockeys have mounted their Horses, and the next call is "SWITCH," the partners switch their immediate roles. And, the command "RACING" can only occur when the Jockey is standing on the ground (i.e., they have not mounted their Horse).

As soon as your group has a basic grasp of what's going on, ramp up the pace of your calls. Works a treat.

Variations

- Introduce a little Simon Says into the game. If the "JOCKEYS UP" or "JOCKEYS DOWN" command is repeated two (or more) times in a row, any Horse and Jockey combination that flinches or moves in anticipation of a different call, will be eliminated. If you want to be really tricky, say "UP" or "DOWN" only and see what happens.

- Introduce a "REST" command, which requires the Jockeys to crawl under the legs of their Horses and sit in front of them. Although now appearing as part of the inside circle, these folk are still the 'Jockeys.'

- If you have a particularly athletic group, when the call of "RACING" is given, the Horse piggy-backs the Jockey all the way around the circle. Last to return is eliminated.

HAVE YOU EVER?

Fun way to explore the diversity of experiences that people bring to a group

AT A GLANCE

A person stands in the middle of a circle and asks a "HAVE YOU EVER...?" question in an attempt to lure one or more people from the group to leave their 'spot' so that he or she may steal it.

WHAT YOU NEED

A chair or spot marker for everyone
15 – 20 mins

WHAT TO DO

Either standing on a 'spot' (a shoe works well), or sitting in seats, ask your group to form a circle. One person, without a spot, will start in the centre of the circle. In the beginning, I like to be this person.

The mission for the person in the centre (the 'Questioner') is to encourage people to leave their seats, so that he or she may steal one for the next round. They do this by asking a question that is prefaced with "HAVE YOU EVER....?" and continue to describe an experience. But whatever the experience, the Questioner must be able to answer 'yes' to his or her own question. So for example, I could ask "HAVE YOU EVER STOOD AT THE LIP OF AN ACTIVE VOLCANO?" because I have – Mt Ruapahu, New Zealand, just for the record! But I could not ask, "HAVE YOU EVER WON A MILLION DOLLARS?" because I haven't. Well, at least not yet.

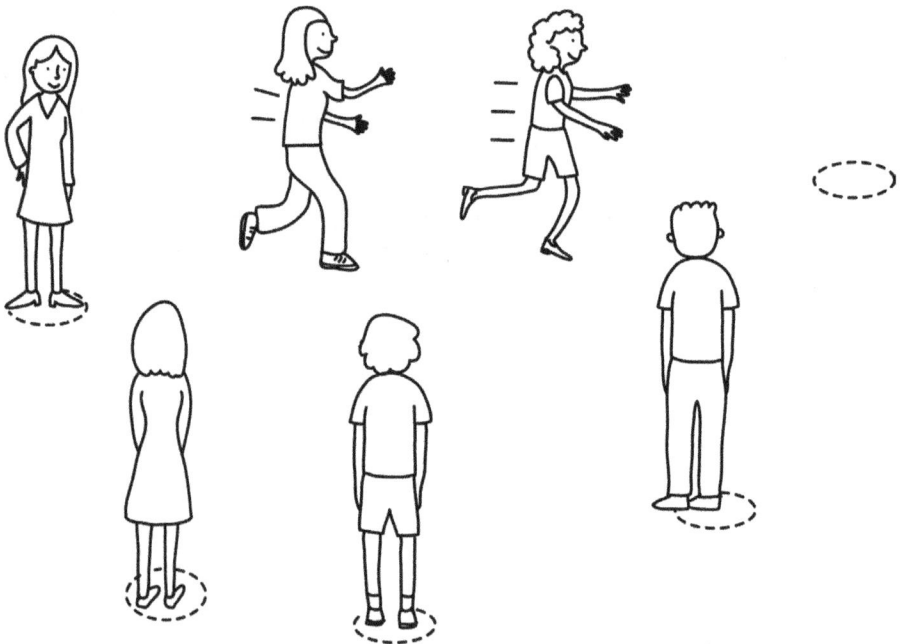

So, the Questioner issues forth their enquiry, and usually, one or more people in the group will think to themselves "Yes, I've done that." Next, explain that everyone who thinks this is invited to leave the safety of their seat, and dart across the circle to find another empty seat. Of course, if seven people get up, there will be eight people looking for a seat (including the Questioner), so someone will miss out – this person will be the next Questioner.

It's a good idea to ask people to think of a question prior to getting caught in the middle and having to say something as profound as , "... UMMM." Also, encourage your group to think of questions a little more creative than "HAVE YOU EVER BRUSHED YOUR TEETH?" This will surely cause lots of movement, but it's rarely fun nor as revealing as "HAVE YOU EVER TOUCHED A GLACIER?" or "WALKED ON A BED OF NAILS?"

You will learn some amazing stuff about people, but remind them that Challenge by Choice still reigns. A person may have, in fact, done the thing that the Questioner has asked, but if they do not feel comfortable 'owning up to it,' they do not have to move, let alone indicate that they had even contemplated it.

I like to honour those freaky folks who pose a question, only to discover that they are the only ones in the group who can respond with a Yes. For example, " BEEN HIT BY LIGHTNING?" and "... ROLLED AN AMBULANCE?" immediately come to mind. In these cases, I invite everyone in the circle to stand, applaud for a few moments, and sit back down. Of course, the Questioner must now think of another question. If anyone gets stuck in the centre and can't think of a good question, or simply doesn't want to be there, they may ask for a volunteer to swap with them.

Variations

- Narrow the scope of your questions such as "HAVE YOU EVER..... AT SCHOOL?," or "HAVE YOU EVER..... WITH YOUR FAMILY?" This strategy will also prevent some groups from thinking up saucy questions when the gambit is very wide.

- Everyone has a 'spot' and anyone can ask "HAVE YOU EVER...?" at any time. In this case, everyone to whom the question applies is invited into the centre to join in a rousing chorus of – Slap-Slap (of thighs), Clap-Clap (of hands), Click-Click (of fingers), "YEAAAHHHHH" (sung gloriously). They all return to their spots and another person gets up with their "HAVE YOU EVER...?,' and so on.

- Prepare a long list of 'Have You Ever?' questions in advance. Read them out to your group, asking each person to score a point for every experience that they have had. Most points wins.

CHIC-A-BOOM

A cool little energiser you can dance and sing to!

AT A GLANCE

A group song and dance that invites people to gradually groove into the centre of the circle.

WHAT YOU NEED

5 – 10 mins

WHAT TO DO

Stand with your group as part of a circle, and teach them these groovy moves. With index fingers, point up into the sky alternating thrusts of each hand to a beat, i.e., left hand up, then right hand up, etc. Now, something similar, but point down with alternate thrusts towards the ground. Next, point your fingers to the left in and out, in and out, as you take little rocking steps to the left. And finally, point your fingers to the right, in and out, in and out as you're taking jaunty little rocking steps to the right.

Okay, as you can tell, it's all in the delivery, but you've got the moves. Taking a big breath, let's set the moves to the chorus:

"….AAAAND, UP CHIC-A-BOOM, CHIC-A-BOOM, CHIC-A-BOOM.

AND DOWN CHIC-A-BOOM, CHIC-A-BOOM, CHIC-A-BOOM.

TO THE LEFT, CHIC-A-BOOM, CHIC-A-BOOM, CHIC-A-BOOM.

TO THE RIGHT, CHIC-A-BOOM, CHIC-A-BOOM, CHIC-A-BOOM."

At this point, with attitude just dripping off you, strut into the centre of

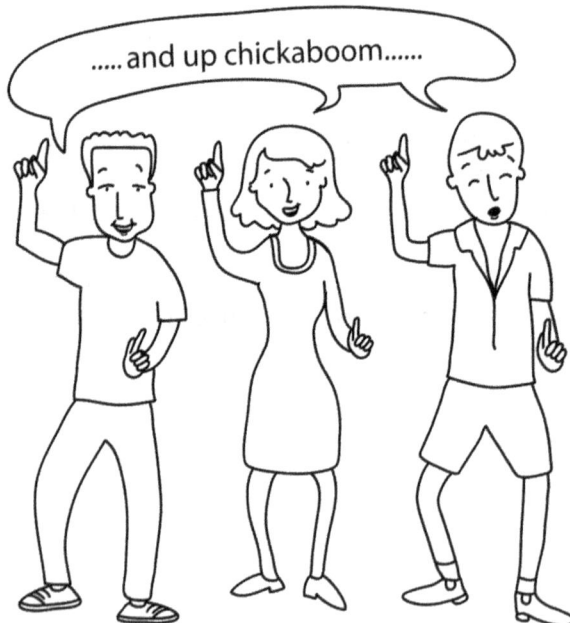

..... and up chickaboom......

the circle, look someone directly in the eyes and launch into:

"HEY THERE (USE THEIR NAME), YOU'RE A REAL COOL CAT.

YOU'VE GOTTA LOT OF THIS, AND YOU'VE GOTTA LOT OF THAT.

SO, COME ON IN AND GET DOWN......"

Who could resist such an invitation? This is your cue to side up to this person, take their arm in yours and lead them into the centre of the circle. Then, you, your new cool cat, and everyone still standing in the circle thinking

"When am I going to be dragged in?" will launch into a medley of the 'Chic-A-Boom' chorus replete with groovy moves and spunk. The up, down, left and right pointing of hands accompanies the chic-a-booms beat-box style. Once you have sung the verse through, every person in the centre (it doubles with every verse) will turn to another standing in the circle and start all over again.

Two begets four, four begets eight, and within four or five verses, you've got everyone in the circle having a great time. Do it for thirty-three verses, and you'll have the whole world "gettin' on down!"

Variation

Do it in reverse, with everyone starting in the centre, and slowly everyone joining the circle.

SAMURAI

An engaging warm-up no matter how many people you've got

AT A GLANCE
Positioned in the centre of a group of people standing in a circle, a 'Samurai' will swing his or her magic sword in one of two ways to cause people to either duck their heads or jump up, lest they be eliminated.

WHAT YOU NEED
Two magic swords, or other enchanted foils
15 – 20 mins

WHAT TO DO
This exercise will largely owe its success to how much you are prepared to 'ham it up.' Inject a ton of life, enthusiasm and commitment into your character, and you WILL become the Samurai.

Ask your group to form a ring around you, standing at least 4 to 5 metres (14 – 17') away from you in the centre. Introduce yourself as the Master Samurai (you may even hear the clang of gongs in the background). Alert your group to the fact that you are wearing a belt, indeed a Black Belt. As you invite everyone to look down at their own waist, you note that they wear only a lowly White Belt. Pity.

Next, explain the mysterious powers you hold over your Samurai sword. When you swish your sword high

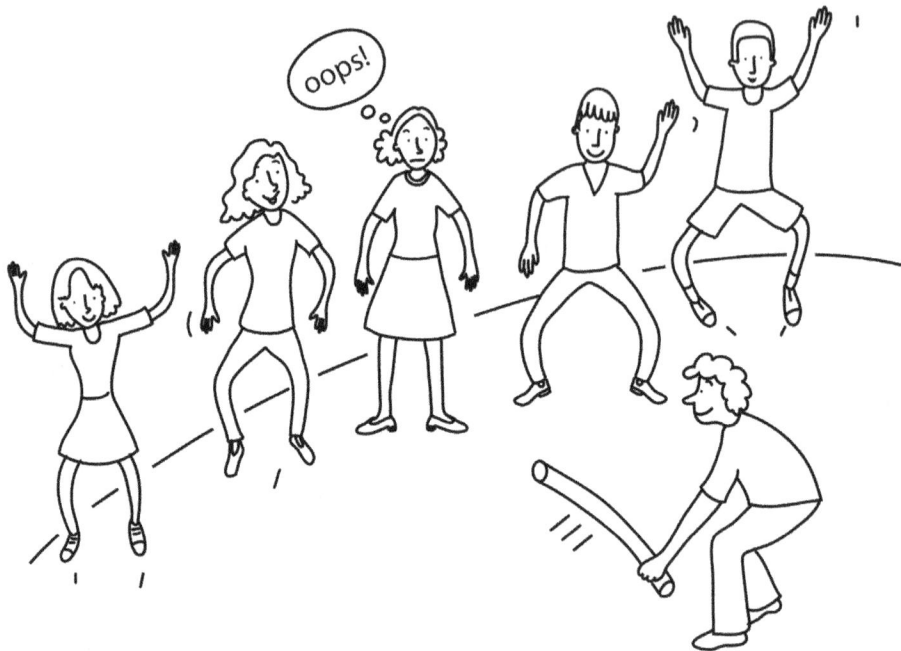

through the air (parallel to the ground) at head height, it will cut people's heads off. Yet, when it is slashed low through the air at knee height, it will cut people's legs off! Happily, describe to your group that they can avoid losing their head by simply ducking their heads and bending down, and may avoid losing their legs by jumping on the spot into the air.

Naturally, the sword does not actually reach nor touch anyone throughout this exercise – just figured I should mention that in case you're wondering! Yet, as powerful as the sword is, there can only be high or low swishes, and the sword only affects those whom are in the path of its arc, i.e., if the sword is swished past or pointed towards a person, only they are affected.

Now to the fun. The Master's clear objective is to eliminate everyone in the circle, by slashing this way and that, slicing heads and chopping knees. Lowly White Belts attempt to remain in the game as long as possible.

You start by respecting the ancient Samurai tradition, and bow to the four corners of the circle, inviting each person to bow back to you. The Master will then start slashing away, making a variety of long and short arcs of his or her sword around the circle. If a White Belt is too slow, or simply ducks when jumping would have been the thing to do, or vice versa, he or she is asked to sit down where they were standing. Last person standing, is invited to assume the role of the Master in the next round.

Note: it really expands the fun if you add audible grunts, shrieks and shrills as the sword is wielded throughout the activity.

Variation

Enter the Kamikaze. Place a second, unused sword in the centre adjacent to the Master. At any time, a person who has been eliminated is entitled to sneak up and snatch the second sword, and challenge the Master to a surprise duel. Following protocols, the two face off, bow, and then engage in mortal combat. The first to tag the other below the knee with the sword is the new Master Samurai. If the challenger wins, everyone is back in the game, and the challenger becomes the new Samurai. However, if the Master wins, the challenger suffers a histrionic death, and must claw his or her way back to the circle.

THE WAVE

Perfect for any circle of very strong chairs

AT A GLANCE

A person, standing in the middle of a group of people seated on chairs, will attempt to sit in the one empty chair before one of the two people sitting on either side of it slide into it.

WHAT YOU NEED

Set of very sturdy chairs (without arm rests), one for every person.
10 – 15 mins

WHAT TO DO

I love this game. It works up a sweat quicker than you can say "Unique New York" six times. But, and it's a BIG But, make sure your chairs are of good, solid, sturdy stock. I have to admit to breaking a few in my time when my eyes for FUNN were bigger than my estimation of costly repairs!

Invite your group to sit on a chair that is part of a perfect circle. By this I mean, no corners, no straight lines, a lovely

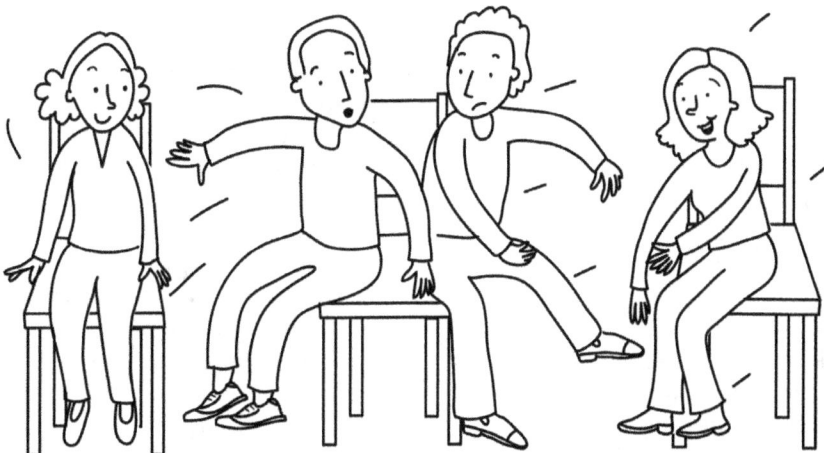

360 degree circle of chairs. Position the chairs so that the legs of one are touching the closest legs of its neighbours.

One person will start, by leaving their seat, causing it to be empty. Strange as it may sound, their goal now is to try to sit back in that empty seat. Or, indeed, any empty seat. You see, as I will explain, at any time a seat is empty, one of the two people sitting beside it will be impelled to slide on to it thereby causing a new seat to become vacant, thus starting the process of someone moving into this newly-created vacant seat. A 'wave' will quickly develop as a series of people (seated together one after the other) shift their position to the left, or to the right.

Of course, during all of this, the empty-nester is trying to find his or her way into a seat. Missed attempts, sitting on laps, and bountiful laughter will result, guaranteed.

When an empty seat is finally filled, one of the two people sitting directly next to the person who filled it (depending on the direction that the wave was travelling) will leave their seat, and the game starts over. Continue until you or your group is exhausted.

Variations

- Allow anyone to reverse the direction of the 'wave' at any time, by faking a move into the vacant seat, but at the last second, deciding to return from whence they came.
- With really large groups, invite several people to vacate their seats. There should be a vacant seat for every person standing in the middle.
- As above, but invite anyone at anytime to leave their seat in an attempt to find another seat. Utter chaos, but pure unadulterated FUNN.

EVERYBODY'S IT

One of the most classic tag games of all time

AT A GLANCE

On "GO," each person chases everyone else to claim a tag, aiming to be the last person standing.

WHAT YOU NEED

5 – 10 mins

WHAT TO DO

This tag is dedicated to all those folks out there who, like me, have experienced the ignominy of being It for a long period of time, i.e., you never realised just how long the lunch recess was – every day! Now that I make up the rules, everyone is going to be It!

It's quite simple really. Start by having the group spread throughout your playing space, and say, "GO." This will launch everyone into a frenzy of contest and self-preservation as they try to tag others whilst avoiding being tagged themselves. A compassionate contact made with one's hand on another's

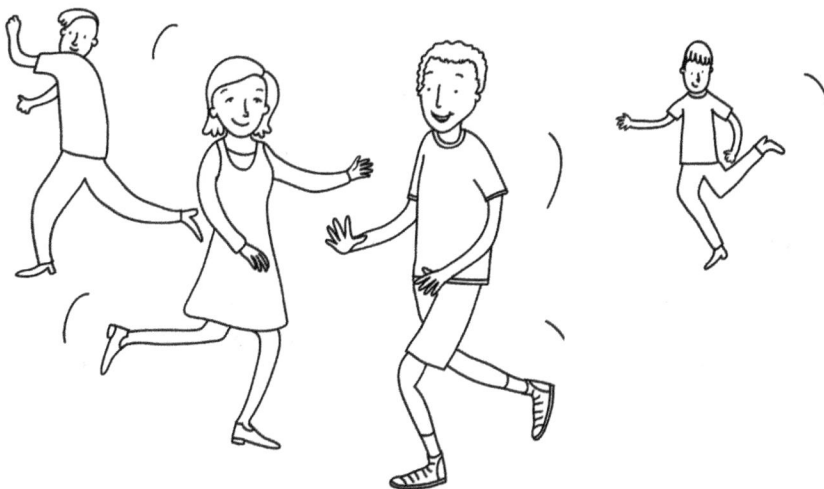

shoulder or back is a sufficient tag. Suggest that as soon as a tag is made, the tagee is obliged to simply crouch down in that spot to indicate to all others that he or she is 'out.' The action continues until the last person remains.

If they are like me, most people will be 'out' within ten seconds – which doesn't necessarily make for a fun time. So, I recommend that you don't give the 'winner' much time to celebrate or be lauded. Instead, surprise everyone with a sudden "GO" and it starts all over again.

Oh, here's my advice for the standard 'What happens when two people tag each other at the same time?' question, which is really the same as, 'I tagged him / her first, but they won't go out' complaint! The people involved have two options. One, they can both declare themselves 'out' and wait for the next round, or two, they can argue for the next minute or two and miss all the fun around them.

Variations

- In the moment of contest, if a person takes a backward step, they are deemed 'out.' Ruthless, I know!

- While crouched down, an 'out' person can tag the passing feet and legs of those folks who still survive (note, stress that only tags are permitted, no grabbing). This action will cause the tagged person to be eliminated as well, and, if you want to introduce a little longevity to the game, entitle the tagger to return to the action.

- Everyone gets three lives. While attempting to tag other people, a person will place a hand on each of the first two areas of their body that have been tagged by another player, and remain in the game until they are tagged a third time. I call this 'Hospital Tag.'

MONARCH

Brilliant tag game that often features strategy, co-operation and team skills

AT A GLANCE

A team, initially represented by one person, attempts to tag every member of the opposing team until every person belongs to his or her team.

WHAT YOU NEED

A soft tossable ball

10 – 20 mins

WHAT TO DO

Having designated a particular playing space for this activity, I often refer to the appointed boundaries as the borders of some nebulous Monarchy in some far off land. I then ask everyone to step inside their 'nation' and subsequently christen them full-blooded Monarchists. Practicing a pompous royal wave is never out of place at this juncture.

Next, I invite one person to volunteer to become the nation's first Republican (or whatever name you wish to give the opposing team). They get to hold the ball, that I refer to as the Royal Sceptre, which they have stolen from the ruling Monarch. The Republican's goal? To convert all of the Monarchists to their cause.

From here on, it's basically a simple tag game, but with just one unique rule. At the very beginning, the lone Republican is the only person who is permitted to run with the ball (otherwise, it may be a very long game). But, as soon as he or she has tagged one of the Monarchists – by tossing the ball and hitting them anywhere below the waist – no one is entitled to move with the ball. That is, if a Republican has the ball in their hands, they can't move their feet. But, happily, a Republican can pass the ball among their team mates.

In case you missed it, once a Monarchist is tagged, they switch loyalty and assist their new Republican friends to tag the remaining Monarchists. Game continues until everyone is a staunch Republican.

Watch as the strategies develop among the Republicans to score a tag. Although clearly a tag game, you may find some value at the end of the activity in discussing and relating the team skills employed during the exercise to the real world.

Got a really large group? I suggest you introduce several 'Republicans' (perhaps one for every 20 to 30 people) each with their own ball.

Variations

- To really highlight the value of strategy and team work, as soon as five Monarchists have been tagged, a Republican is not entitled to move (except for retrieving errant balls). That is, they must remain standing in the spot where they were tagged, although a pivot of one foot is permitted.
- Introduce the rule that the last two remaining Monarchists must be male and female (so that they can re-populate the Monarchist world, of course!).

OCTOPUS TAG

A tag in which everyone eventually becomes It

AT A GLANCE

A group attempts to move from one side of an area to the other as many times as possible without being tagged. Upon being tagged, a person will switch roles and attempt to tag others.

WHAT YOU NEED

10 – 20 mins

WHAT TO DO

Looking for another 'wear-them-out' exercise? This is it.

Start your group on one side of a large hall or playing field. Their goal is to run to the opposite side and back as many times as possible without being tagged. Explain that in the beginning, only one person will be a designated 'Tagger,' and he or she will be roaming about somewhere in the middle of the area.

On "GO," the chase begins. Let's say that on the first pass from one side to the other, the Tagger only manages to tag three people from the group. This may seem like a loss – when you consider that dozens more escaped – but the Tagger has now recruited three more people to his or her cause. Much like an octopus, eight arms for tagging are better than two! The tagging team now accounts for four people.

However, unlike the Tagger – who is always entitled to move anywhere within the area – all new taggers must remain on the spot where they were tagged. They are entitled to pivot on one foot from this 'spot,' but otherwise, their movements are restricted.

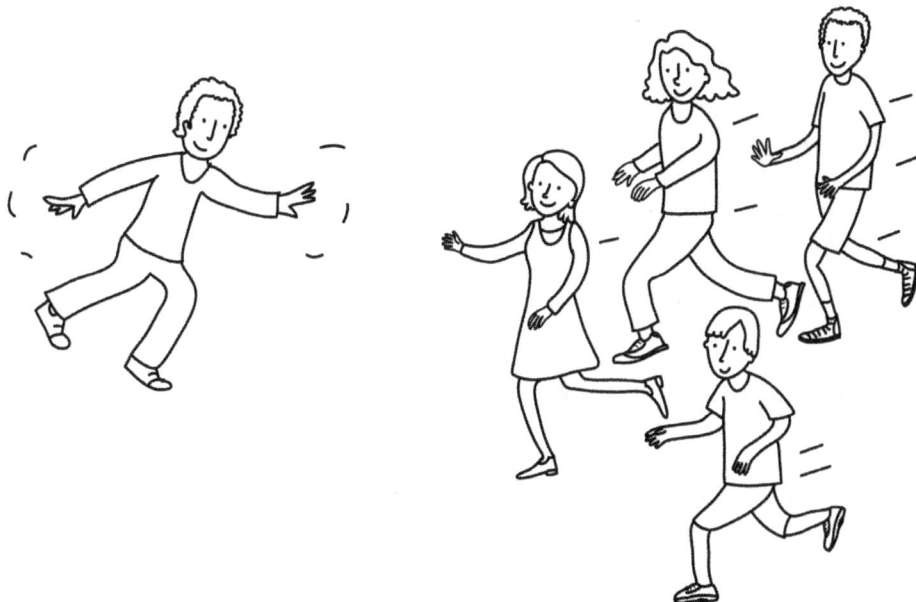

So, the group continues to pass from one side to the other. Each time the group may (or may not) lose one or more of its number to assume tagging-on-the-spot roles. The game continues until everyone is tagged.

Variations

- As above, but the newly tagged must sit on the floor / ground where they were tagged as they attempt to tag others in the group passing them.
- One person from the 'tagging' team can announce how the group must cross the area for the next pass, e.g., skipping, hop on one leg, run sideways, etc.
- Announce that the group's goal is to preserve two people at the end, one male and one female (or two other distinctions of any kind). This variation will involve a lot more strategy to ensure that the two 'types' of people are kept safe at the very end.

MAD CHEFS

One of the most purposeful and enduring tag games I know

AT A GLANCE
Within a time limit, individuals approach as many 'good chefs' as they can to write a food on their paper plate, whilst avoiding a group of 'mad chefs' who are intent on striking the foods off the plate.

WHAT YOU NEED
A pen for every 5 people
Bunch of paper plates
Chef hats and aprons (optional)
15 – 30 mins

WHAT TO DO
Nominate approximately one person (or staff member) for every five people in your group to be a 'chef' – half of whom you will identify as 'good' and the other half as 'mad' (think, bad). Arm each chef with a pen. Using some method (e.g., signs, hats, or different coloured aprons) to help participants identify which chef is good or bad, introduce each team of chefs with a flourish to generate the obligatory cheers and hisses from your group.

Now, hand a paper plate to every other person in your group and explain that their goal is to 'collect' as much food on their plate as is possible within, say, 5 to 10 minutes. Explain that foods will be added to a person's plate when they visit a good chef, while (boo, hiss) they will lose a food item every time a mad chef catches them. Yes, this is every inch a tag game.

Kick off the game by asking all of the chefs to spread like the wind, and distribute themselves evenly throughout the playing area. On "GO," everyone will race about willy-nilly trying to locate the good chefs, while at the same time, trying to avoid the mad chefs. Good chefs are welcome to stay put in one spot (but they can move about to increase the fun), while the mad chefs will raise a good sweat very quickly.

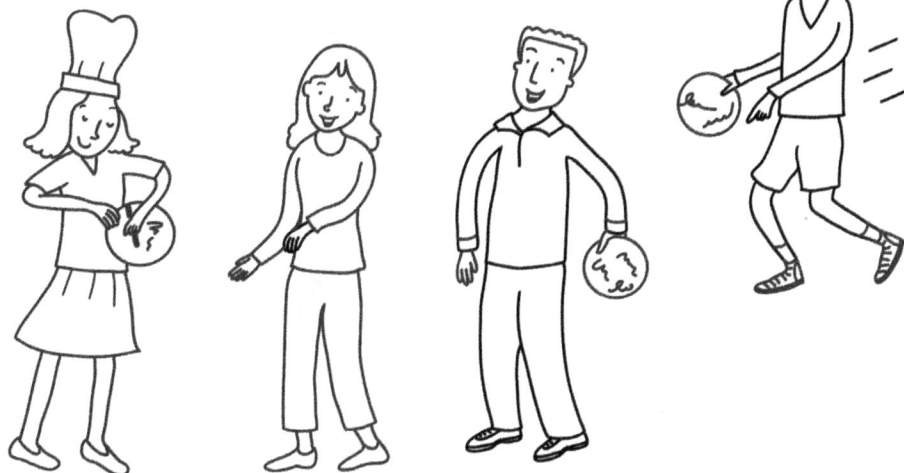

When a good chef is located, a person will stand in line, and wait their turn to have a food (any food, it doesn't matter) written onto their plate. Standing in line is a good thing because it means that they are 'safe' from being tagged. However, you should set a maximum number that can be allowed to be in line to be considered 'safe.' Three or four people seems to work pretty well – the smaller your group, the smaller the queue. So, if a mad chef approaches a line of, let's say, five people standing in front of a good chef (and the limit is three people), the fourth and fifth stand-in-liners can be tagged.

Now, when a mad chef tags a participant (note, I suggest 'tag,' not rugby tackle), the chef is entitled to strike off one of the foods written on the plate. To be fair, a mad chef should not hover around a good chef, ready to tag a recently food-laden participant – but it is fun.

At the end of, say, two or more short rounds (take a water break between each round), gather everyone and count up the number of foods written on each plate. The person(s) with the most foods, wins! Yum.

Variations

- Establish several 'teams' in advance, before releasing the hungry hordes.

- The good and bad 'chefs' are not announced (i.e., their identity is kept secret at first) and are fixed in one position on the floor. The chefs (particularly, the mad chefs) can only pivot on one foot from this position in order to reach and tag a passing participant.

ASTEROIDS

A classic tossable tag game that offer tons of variations

AT A GLANCE

A person attempts to eliminate everyone else in their group, while also avoiding elimination, by throwing soft tossable items to hit others below the waist.

WHAT YOU NEED

A soft tossable item for each person
10 – 20 mins

WHAT TO DO

On paper, this could read like 'just another tag game.' If it does, then go back to the front of this book and re-read the article Your Approach is Everything on page 14. It's all about your approach. Hence, this remains one of my top sixty activities!

Having passed a soft tossable to everyone (e.g., fleece-ball, rolled up sock), ask your group to bunch in real close to the centre of your playing space. With tongue firmly planted in the side of your cheek, explain that this activity is really just a representation of how the universe was created – with the 'big bang' (with apologies to all my creationist friends out there). So, the game starts with everyone leaning in to create the biggest, fluffiest soft tossable / fleece-ball / whatever, and then on "GO" will throw their items high into the air.

At this point, people will quickly scatter and grab one or more tossables, and start to piff them at one another. The idea is, if someone is hit anywhere

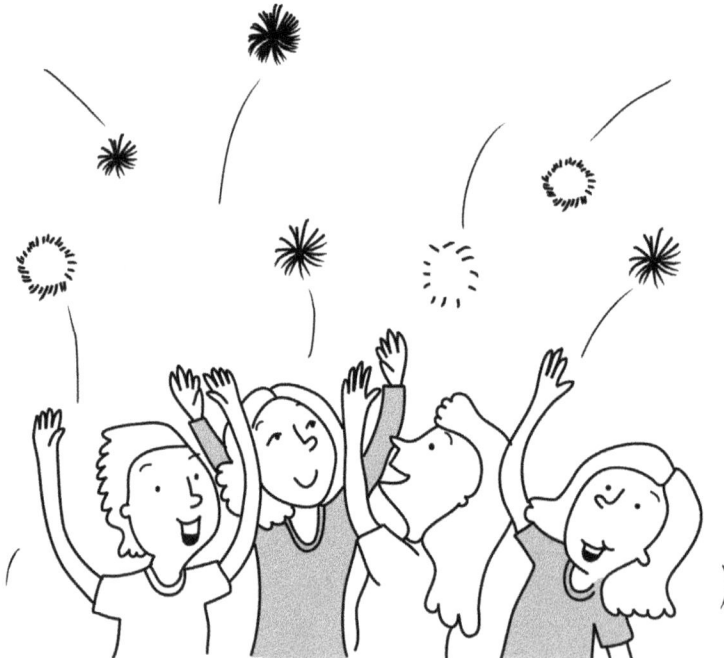

below their waist, they are eliminated, and asked to simply crouch down on the spot where they were hit (mindful of the action around them).

The first round normally takes about 20 seconds, give or take a few. Not much fun if you were the first to go out. So, I then introduce the 'Asteroid Rule.' An eliminated person is now entitled to come back into the fray if they can grab a passing tossable (aka asteroid) from their crouching position (pivoting on one knee is kosher). Allllright. Bunch on back in, and start again.

Now, the game has longevity – unless of course, you are stuck way out on the edges of the galaxy, and no asteroids are to be seen anywhere. If this is the case, try a variation below.

Variations

- A person who is eliminated may tag (notice I said 'tag' and not grab) the ankle or leg of a passing player. If this occurs, the player and tagger switch roles.

- Or, upon a successful tag, the player must stand still for five seconds while the tagger calls loudly "TARGET, TARGET" to get the attention of other players. If the tagged player is hit with a tossable within the five seconds, he or she switches roles with the tagger. If not, the player is free to roam again.

CLOTHES-PEG TAG

Excellent for stimulating lots of energy and action

AT A GLANCE
Armed with a swag of clothes-pegs (clothes-pins), a person will aim to attach as many pegs as possible onto other people, while also trying to dodge extra pegs being pinned on them.

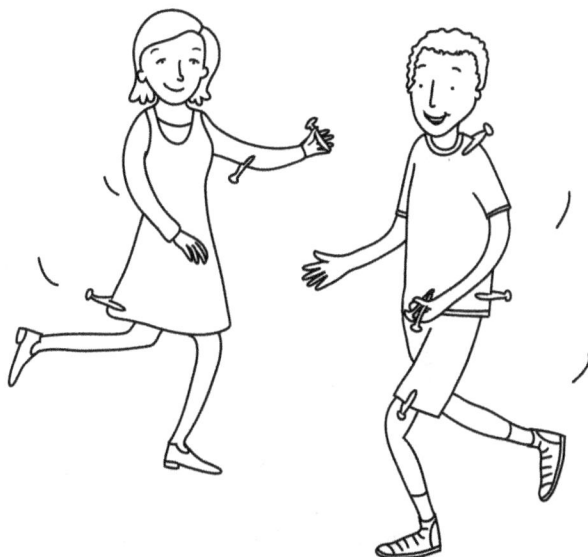

WHAT YOU NEED
A big bag of clothes-pegs
10 – 15 mins

WHAT TO DO
Collect as many pegs as would supply 4 to 8 pegs per person. Then distribute this same number of pegs to everyone in your group, and ask them to pin

them onto their clothing somewhere. The pegs need to be accessible, that is, somewhere on the upper torso, preferably on the back, front or arms of the clothing.

I doubt you will need boundaries for this activity, because the fun is always in the centre, but go ahead and set them if necessary. On "GO," everyone aims to take as many of their own pegs off their clothing (one at a time), and attach them to other people's clothing. To be clear, all pegs must remain on a person's clothing except for the one they are trying to attach to someone else. Naturally, it's not a one-way street; often when a person is not looking, they don't suspect that someone is slyly pinning a peg on their back.

Run the game for as long as you feel there is energy, then stop and count each person's stash of pegs. Pretty simple, the person with the least wins.

Variation

Try it in reverse. Everyone aims to steal as many pegs from others in their group and attach them to their clothing.

STRIKER

Ideal run-them-until-they're-ragged wide game

AT A GLANCE
Two teams compete to hit a beach ball with their open hands across a wide, open playing area in the direction of their designated goal.

WHAT YOU NEED
One (preferably two or more) inflatable beach balls
Wide, open space
10 – 20 mins

WHAT TO DO
Small areas just don't work with this activity. The bigger and wider the better.

Allocate your group into two teams. Feel free to identify each team somehow (e.g., wear different coloured tops, socks-up/socks-down, etc), but generally it's not necessary. Next, designate an area for each team to represent their goal. The goals should be at least 50 metres apart. I normally lay a rope or indicate an imaginary line between two points as sufficient. If playing inside, opposing walls are perfect.

Now, introduce a fully blown (and hopefully sturdy) beach ball. The object for each team is to strike or hit the ball – with an open hand – in the direction of their goal so that it passes over the goal line (or hits the wall) as many times as possible. The team with the most goals wins. No one is permitted to hold or grasp the ball, otherwise, there are no possession rules, fouls, or free-kicks. Once the ball is launched into the air to signify the start, play begins. When a goal is scored, the ball is returned to the centre to be launched high into the air again.

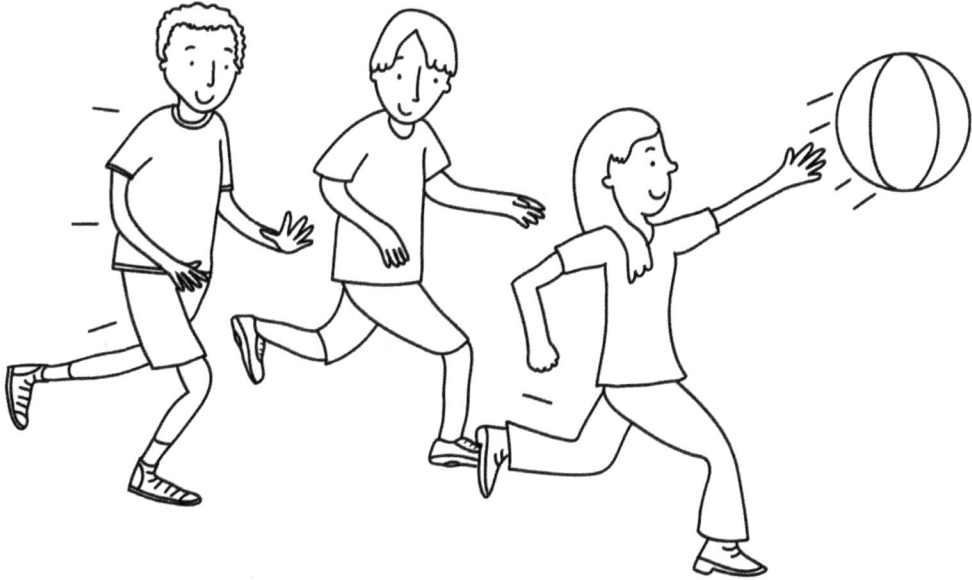

Once this basic concept has been grasped and a few goals have been scored, you may notice that not everyone follows the ball to remain active. If so, introduce a second or third ball to whip up a little more energy, not to mention, a lot more people. This game can tire people out quickly, so play for five to ten minutes, take a break, and then swap goals to play a second half.

You could use any softish ball, but I have found that the weightlessness and unpredictability of a beach ball is a great leveller when it comes to sporting prowess. A beach ball can make even the coolest, most athletic dude or dudette look like a klutz.

Word of warning, borne from experience – always keep a few spare beach balls handy, because they do break. And, don't try this outside on a windy day. In no time flat, you'll have everyone running for the ball three blocks away.

Variation

Try three or four teams, all competing to strike the ball through their designated goal.

KING'S TREASURE

Another wonderful 'run-them-until-they're-ragged' exercise

AT A GLANCE

The members of a small group attempt to steal as many items of 'treasure' from the lair of every other small group within a set time limit.

WHAT YOU NEED

As many soft tossable items as you can get

4 buckets

10 – 15 mins

WHAT TO DO

Separate your group into four even teams, and allocate them a particular corner area of your hall or playing field. Hand each team a bucket filled with an equal number of soft tossable items, such as fleece-balls, squeaky toys, rolled-up socks, etc, and ask them to place them somewhere accessible within their area.

Explain that this exercise will occur over several rounds. The object for each team is to collect as many items in their buckets as possible, more than any other team. They do this by simply running to the area of any small team and 'stealing' no more than one item at a time and returning to place it into their own bucket. There is no limit to the number of people from a team who can be involved in stealing at the same time.

Not many rules, other than to alert people to the fact that there will be a lot of activity between the areas, so each person should be aware of other people and be safety conscious. Also, no one is permitted to guard the buckets. Every bucket is free game.

And, "GO." Watch the frenzy. There are few activities that work harder at exhausting participants. Allow two minutes for the first round, do a count and announce the interim results. Play two or more rounds (with short rests in between), depending on your group's level of energy and enthusiasm for the treasure, accumulate the results and congratulate the winning team.

Variations

- Start with all the items in the centre of the playing space, a.k.a. the King's Treasure.

- Limit each team to one or two people who can steal items at any point in time.

- Use balloons instead of soft tossables.

WATER WORLD

Great fun, and simply one of the best excuses for a water-fight!

AT A GLANCE
Armed with a number of water-filled cups, a team aims to fill their bucket with as much water as possible, while avoiding the spoiling tactics of the opposition.

WHAT YOU NEED
A cup for every second person (avoid disposable cups where possible)

Several regular sized buckets

Several large barrels filled with water

Water hose to continuously fill the barrels

20 – 30 mins

WHAT TO DO
To prepare, position one (or more) empty buckets at one end of your field, and one (or more) large barrels at the other end. It's not an exact science, but try to space the buckets and the barrels at least 100 metres (330') apart. Fill the barrels with water, and keep the hose handy.

Separate your group into two teams, and elect one team to start in defence (protector of the buckets) and the other in offence (holder of the cups). The offence – armed with empty cups – will start by filling their cups with water from the large barrels. Then, as swiftly and gingerly as they can, race their water-laden cups across the field – avoiding the spoiling tactics of the protectors (that is, getting tagged) – and empty the contents of their cup (if any) into a bucket. The objective is simple – the team with the most water in a bucket at the end of the game, wins! Play a round of say 10 minutes each, and then swap roles, i.e., the protectors

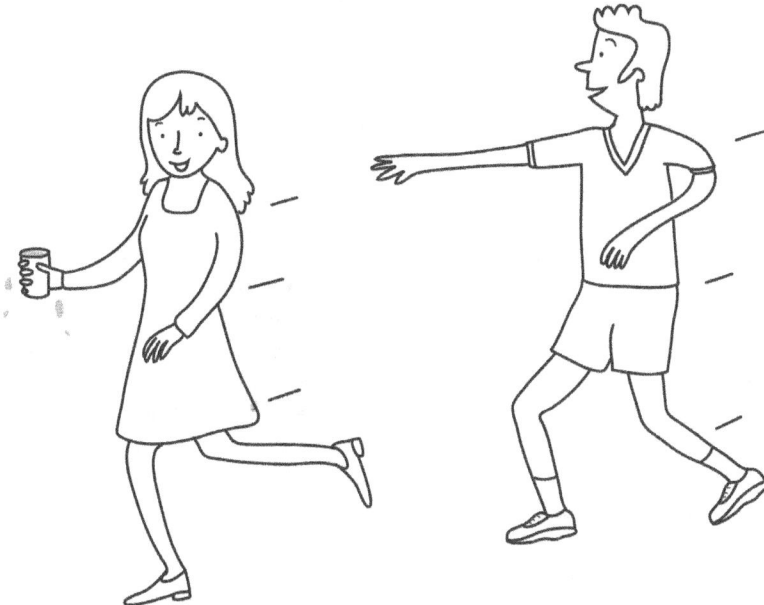

now take the cups, and vice versa.

A few rules to make the chase worthwhile:

- The protectors must maintain a distance of at least five metres (17′) from the water-filled barrels and the buckets (this gives the 'cup team' a sporting chance, at least in the beginning).

- When members of the 'cup team' are tagged by the defence (no rugby tackles please), they must pour the water in their cup over their heads.

- If members of the 'cup team' suspect that they are about to be tagged, they can immediately stop the proceedings and choose to do one of two things:

  - Pour the water on their heads (i.e., they were going to get tagged anyway); or

  - Throw the water at the annoying protector.

Like I said, it's a great excuse for a water fight.

Variation

Set up barrels and buckets for each team at opposing ends, and equip every person with a cup. Now every one is a cupster and a protector at the same time.

CAPTURE THE FLAGS

A wonderfully exhausting variation of a 'golden-oldie'

AT A GLANCE

One team of people attempt to steal all of their opponent's flags, before their opponent steals all of theirs, all the time working to avoid being tagged and / or eliminated.

WHAT YOU NEED

20 flags or other fancy items
Bunch of soft tossable items
2 buckets
20 – 30 mins

WHAT TO DO

If you did not grow up with the 20th century classic 'Capture the Flag,' the first thing you need to know is that you need lots of playing space. And, in this brilliant variant, you will also need lots of flags.

Identify a large area and divide it neatly in half. One half of the space belongs to one half of your group, and vice versa. This is their home turf, and is considered 'safe.' Now, place ten easily identifiable flags and a bucket at the rear of each safe area. The bigger and wider your space, the better. Arm each team with a bunch of soft tossables, such as fleece-balls, and you are ready to explain the rules.

Upon an agreed signal, each team will attempt to enter the space of their opponent, try to steal one or more of

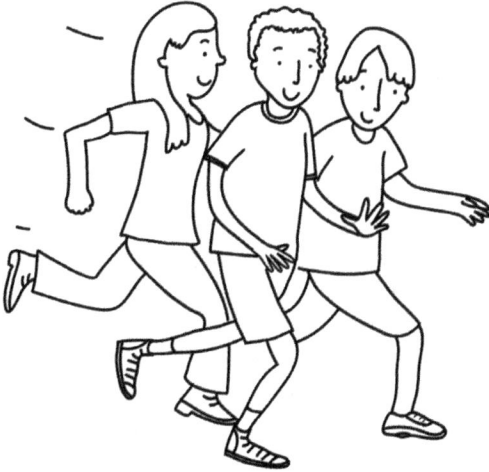

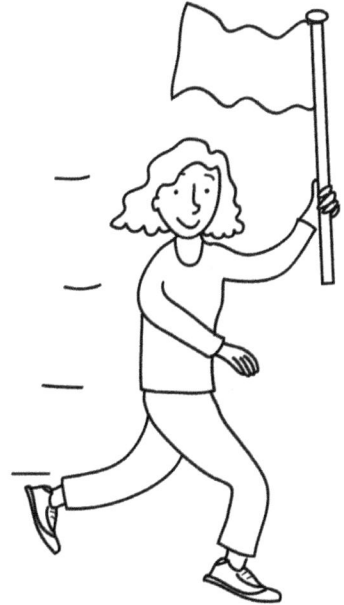

their opponent's flags, return to their safe area and place them in their bucket. One person can only steal one flag at a time. The first team to recover all ten flags, or eliminate all of their opponents, wins. Which raises the question, how does someone get eliminated?

A person may be eliminated by being (a) tagged when they are in their opponent's safe area, or (b) hit by a soft tossable when they are in their own safe area. If someone has successfully stolen a flag, but is eliminated before they can place the flag into their team's bucket, the flag must be dropped immediately and may be reclaimed by either team. Being eliminated simply means enjoying the action from the sidelines.

Strategy clearly plays a role in this activity, so feel free to allow each team some time before and during the contest (if you give them several five minute rounds) to plan their attack. But keep it light, it's a game remember. It's nice to win, but this ain't warfare.

Variations

- To keep more people active for longer, allow eliminated people to return to the fray after one or two minutes. So, in effect, the team to successfully steal all of their opponent's flags first wins.

- House eliminated participants for each team in a 'Jail' situated somewhere in their opponent's safe area. These folk can be released if a member of their team 'breaks into' the jail and tags them without being eliminated.

ULTIMATE HAND BALL

A fun variation of an old school-yard favourite

AT A GLANCE

Each person attempts to eliminate other people in their group by striking a ball so that it hits them anywhere below the knee, while also dodging the ball to avoid being hit.

WHAT YOU NEED

Several 20 cm (8") rubber-coated foam balls

10 – 20 mins

WHAT TO DO

You first learned to play Dodge Ball or Bombardment at school, right? Enough said. This ain't the same game. This is Ultimate Hand Ball.

The game works best if you can play in a large arena or hall, because four walls will prevent the balls from escaping. However, if you don't have a big hall, take a look at one of the later variations.

Ask your group to stand anywhere within the defined playing space, and explain that there are no teams, i.e., basically, it's every person for him or her self. Introduce one or more soft, rubber-coated balls and explain that whenever someone is hit or touched below the knee by one of the balls, they are deemed 'out of the game.'

The game continues until one person is left standing.

There are several rules which will assist you to keep the game safe, fun and fair:

- All hits of the ball must occur with an open hand.
- A direct hit, or one that occurs after one or more bounces, will eliminate anyone it touches.
- If someone is touched by a rolling ball, he or she is also eliminated.
- A direct hit that results in a ball being caught (without a bounce) will cause the 'hitter' to be eliminated.

Naturally, with two or more balls in play at any time, the action can be quite intense. To give the game a little longevity, announce that if a ball is caught (on the full), the 'hitter' is eliminated as per the rules, but, everyone who is 'out' can return to the game.

Just one word of caution – alert your group to the tendency of some who like to 'wind up' before hitting a ball. As people often crowd around a ball as it approaches, it is possible for someone to whack another as they swing their hand high before attempting to strike the ball.

Variations

- Play on a basketball court (with hoops drawn). If a ball is caught by anyone who has been eliminated (as they stand on the sidelines), they are entitled to take a shot at the closest goal from where they were standing. If they score, everyone is back in the game.

- If outside, designate a large circle in which to play. Retrieve any stray balls as they occur, and explain that only hits made inside the circle are 'official.'

- Separate your group into two teams. One team stands to form a giant circle, while the other team plays ball on the inside. As playing team members are eliminated, they join the circle team. If a ball penetrates the circle's perimeter, a member from the circle team may strike the ball back into play, eliminating an opponent perchance! Swap teams at half time.

CIRCLE THE CIRCLE

A circle activity that encourages problem-solving and co-operation

AT A GLANCE

A group of people standing in a circle holding hands work together to manoeuvre a hula hoop – that has been threaded over people's arms – around the circle.

WHAT YOU NEED

Several hula hoops
15 – 30 mins

WHAT TO DO

Ask your group to stand in a circle, and for each person to hold the hands of their partners. Look around, and observe that some people like to hold their hands in a particular way – stereotypically speaking, men like to hold hands with their palms facing back, whereas women tend to hold with their palms facing forward! It means absolutely nothing, of course, but it is interesting!

Having distracted your group's focus for a few moments, casually introduce a hula hoop into the circle, by first releasing one of your partner's hands, poking your hand through the centre of the hoop, and then re-clasping your partner's hand. The hoop should now be resting on the top of your arm or wrist.

At this point, call your group's attention, and challenge them to pass this hoop around the circle, without letting go of their partner's hands, or as much as possible, using their fingers or thumbs to manoeuvre the hoop. Most will either step into it, or poke their heads and upper torsos through. A few will even look at you blankly and wonder how to do it. But people soon catch on.

Once the hoop has travelled its full orbit, allow it to continue on its journey for a second time, then without notice or fanfare, introduce a new hoop, but this time, send it in the opposite direction. Continue to introduce more hoops at appropriate intervals, in different directions to up the challenge. If you have hula hoops of different sizes, pass the larger hoops in one direction, and the smaller hoops the other way to make them easier to pass one another.

Continue this for as long as there is enthusiasm, and you can see people working well together. Or, whenever one poor soul gets lumbered with all of

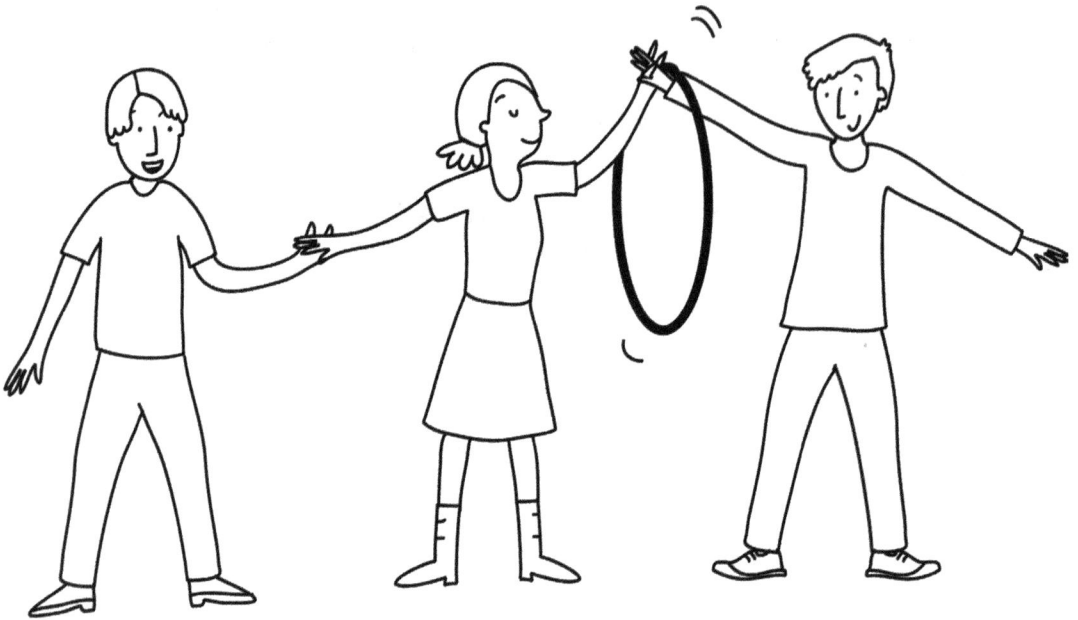

the hoops. A non-threatening warm up and stretch activity, that also features lots of cooperation, problem-solving and fun.

If you have a particularly large group, introduce several hoops into the circle all at once – this will prevent boredom from setting in.

Variations

- Using just one hoop (or two – going in opposite directions – if it's a very large group), set your group the challenge to pass the hoop around the circle as quickly as possible. Time it, and give your group three official attempts with ample time between each to problem solve.

- Rather than, or in addition to, using hula hoops, introduce one or more 'hoops' made of rope (i.e., tie two ends of a short rope together). Rope rings are much more difficult to pass because they are not rigid and often get twisted.

- Introduce several hula hoops into the circle, evenly spaced. The hoops all travel in the same direction. The group aims to pass each hoop more quickly than the one ahead of it so that the two hoops eventually meet. I like to call this one 'Fox and Hound.'

FOUR LETTER WORD

A great mixer as much as a problem-solving activity

AT A GLANCE

Holding a card with a letter of the alphabet written on it, two or more people will combine their letters to form a series of words and / or sentences.

WHAT YOU NEED

Set of 100 alphabet cards
15 – 30 mins

WHAT TO DO

Your first step is to source a set of alphabet cards, or better still, make your own. Model your set on the number of tiles a regular SCRABBLE game gives each letter. Don't have a SCRABBLE set handy? Then look at page 236 as a guide.

Gather your group, and randomly distribute one alphabet card to each person (if you have fewer than 30 people,

distribute two cards per person). From here, you have many options. Here's a few of my favourites in a sequence that has worked for me many times. Ask your group to:

- Form one straight line according to the alphabetical order of the cards. Clearly, this is not a four-letter word, but it gives everyone an idea of what letters are available.

- Form a four-letter word. Aim to involve everyone in a word. If necessary, suggest that already formed four-letter words disband in an attempt to involve everyone in a word.

- With different partners, form a new four-letter word.

- Form a three-letter word, then (after a few minutes) a five-letter word, and finally a six-letter word.

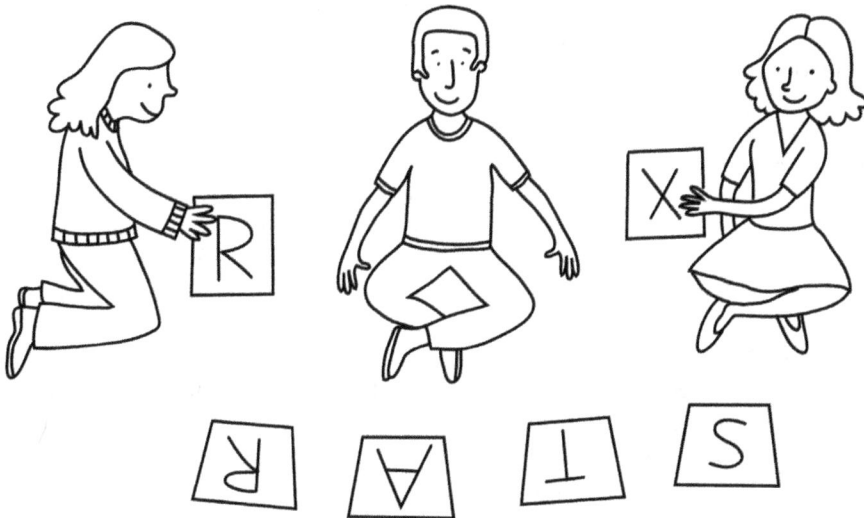

- Invite three or more 'words' (small groups of people), to combine their letters and invent a short sentence or phrase that uses all of the letters, as much as possible. The stunted, half-cocked sentences that develop are often hilarious.

It's up to you if you allow proper nouns and place names, acronyms, etc, as if you were really playing SCRABBLE. However, if this occurs with a 'high performance' group, I would suggest you applaud their efforts and then challenge them to find another solution.

Variations

- Ask your group to form letters, phrases and sentences that follow a theme, such as the values of their organisation, or important team work principles.

- Provide your group with the full 26 letter alphabet, you know, A to Z. Their mission is to use every letter to form a series of words in a format similar to SCRABBLE. That is, a particular letter can be used twice by two words, in the across and down directions. Tough, but doable (if you don't believe me, look at page 236 for one solution). For really large groups, separate into smaller groups, each with their own alphabet.

PAPER PLANE CONTEST

The perfect test for all those paper plane aficionados

AT A GLANCE
Supplied with a sheet of paper, each person attempts to construct a paper plane that will fly the furthest, highest or the longest.

WHAT YOU NEED
A ream of paper
15 – 30 mins

WHAT TO DO
This ain't sixth grade anymore. This is serious. Who can build and fly the best paper plane? Let's find out.

Distribute the sheets of paper, and, perhaps following a brief class in Paper Plane Design 101, let your group at it. This has to be one of those skills that comes with the genes, because only some people profess to have a certain aeronautical expertise when it comes to paper. Yet, you'll be amazed at the results, not to mention the variety of designs and their flight patterns.

Once assembled, herald the start of the competition. Stand everyone along a line, or with their backs to the wall, and let 'em fly. One at a time works best, because then everyone can share in the joy (or despair) of their colleagues' flights. There are three or four common competitions; the longest / furthest flight, the highest flight (hard to measure sometimes), the longest aloft, and the most number of loop-the-loops.

Oh, by the way, let me give you something to aim for. Ken Blackburn is named in the Guinness Book of Records as having recorded the world's longest time aloft for a paper plane, at a whopping 27.6 seconds. Was this guy on the moon or what?

Variations

- Separate your group into small teams of six to eight people, and instruct them to build their best paper plane (one only) to enter into one or more contests. They may have a different design for each level of competition.

- Adding to above, prior to announcing the start of a contest, ask each group to nominate who in their team is the most accomplished paper plane designer. Then ask these 'experts' to swap into another team, and teach this new team what they know. Great way to share the love around. This scenario can also reward you with some wonderful processing points; for example, "How did your group feel to lose its 'expert?' Was it easy for your team to learn from someone else?" etc.

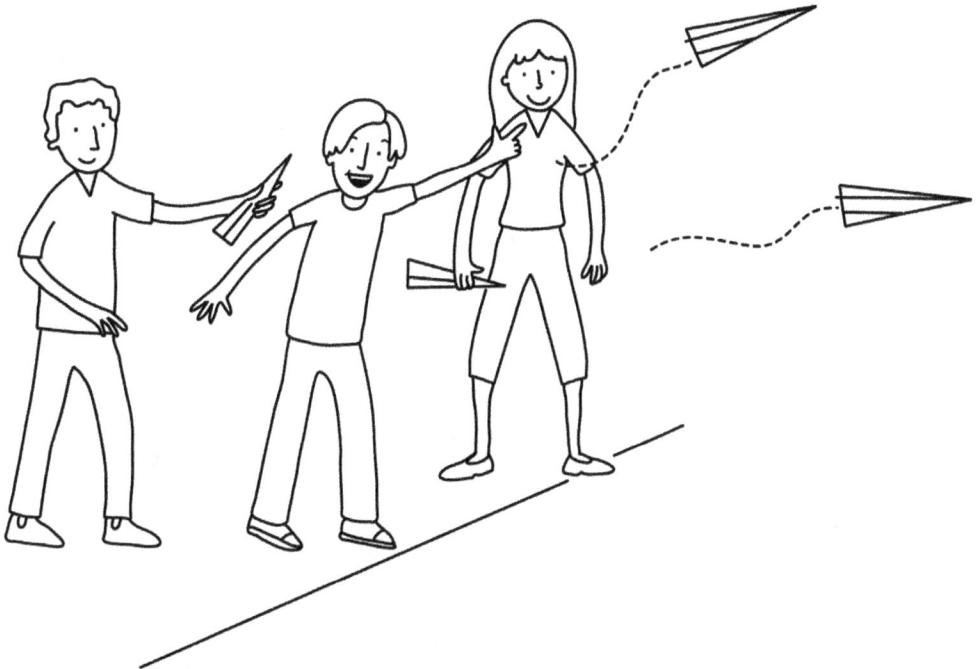

FUNNY WALK

A gradual building up of trust to look silly in front of others

AT A GLANCE

People are invited to walk in the most ridiculous manner they can invent back and forth from one side of a space to the other several times in different configurations.

WHAT YOU NEED

10 – 15 mins

WHAT TO DO

Designate one area from which your group will start, and another to which your group will move. Starting from behind the first line, gather your group and explain that you would like each person to walk independently from here to the other side.

Explain that each person is now invited to walk in a way that no one else has ever walked before. It's a good idea for you to cross the area first playing absolutely full-out, to spark your group's imagination. Then, upon arriving at your destination (having soaked up all the titters along the way), invite everyone else to follow you. Also, to quell any 'people-will-look-at-me' concerns, encourage your group to walk across the area at the same time, or whenever they are ready to go.

Once everyone has crossed, step up the challenge and ask each person to find a partner, and cross back to the other side together, but this time joined somehow physically with the other. Again, this pair must walk in a fashion that has never been seen before. Upon this second crossing, two pairs join forces to form a quad, and repeat the process, each time inventing an all-together-never-been-seen-before walk. As you can guess, the expanding walks culminate in the entire group

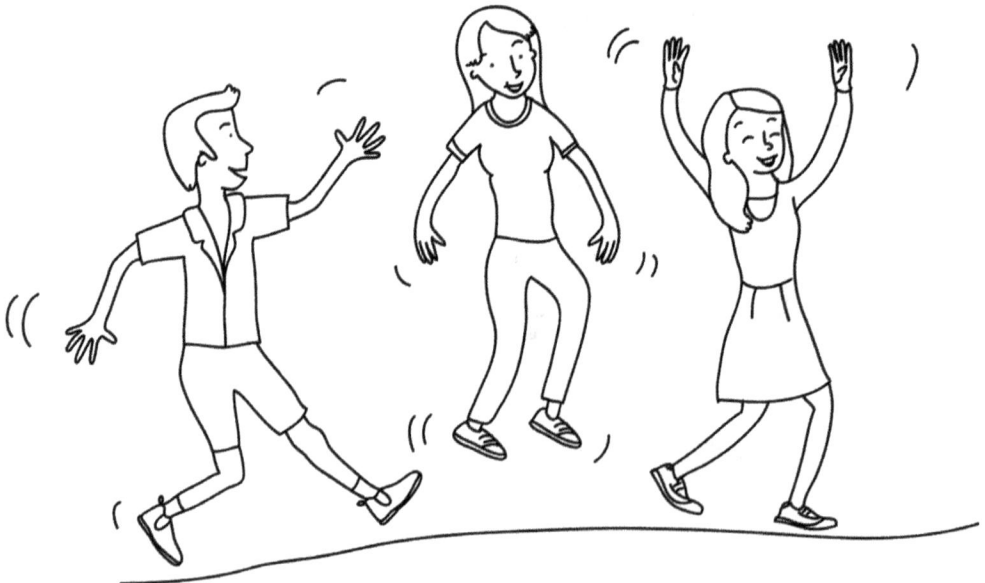

crossing jointly in one final celebratory walk to the finish line.

Does it matter that several people adopt a similar walk? In a word, nuh! It's not the point. Inviting people to mix, solve problems, and laugh together is.

Variation

Adopt this silliness to move a group a long distance, progressing forward about 10 to 20 metres (30 - 60') with each round, until you arrive at your destination.

DRESS ME UPS

A wonderful variation of 'dress ups' that we all loved as kids

AT A GLANCE

A volunteer is 'dressed' by a small group in the most outrageous manner, and then performs a little show for everyone.

WHAT YOU NEED

Trunk of used clothing, hats, accessories, make-up, etc (optional)

20 – 30 mins

WHAT TO DO

Unless you already have pre-assigned groupings, separate your group into teams of about six to eight participants, and allocate one willing staff member, or volunteer participant, to act as the 'mannequin' or 'model' for each team. Then, with all the pomp and pageantry you can muster, announce that each team will have approx 20 minutes (you decide) to dress their mannequin in whatever and however they like. Other than all the clothing, costumes, make-up, etc that they can get their hands on, there are no limits to how they may 'dress' their mannequin – the more bizarre the better.

Allow each small group to prepare / dress in private, and then upon returning to the common meeting area, suggest that the embellishments of each 'model' are kept secret, perhaps using a blanket, until they are finally exposed. As the models shrug off their covers, ask them to give a little cat-walk performance reflecting the spirit of their 'dress.' Expect howls of laughter.

Variations

- Same set-up, but this time, the willing models strip down to their swim-wear (if deemed appropriate), and let their group paint them. Non-toxic, water-based paints are a must, and expect just as much fun, but a whole lot more mess.

- Restrict the items that can be used to 'dress up' a model. For example, use only newspaper, or bath towels, toilet tissue, etc.

PICTIONARY

One of the best large group adaptations of a popular board game around

AT A GLANCE

Taking turns, one person in a small group attempts to draw an object – without using any verbal communication – to help their group identify it as quickly as possible.

WHAT YOU NEED

Sheet(s) of large paper for each small group

Markers / pens for each group

List of 'things' to be drawn

20 – 30 mins

WHAT TO DO

Start by organising your group into smaller teams of about six to eight people, and spread them evenly throughout your area. Issue each group one or more large sheets of paper and pens, and explain the basic rules of the popular board game 'Pictionary.' It's a game that many people will already know, but here are the basics:

- One person draws something that the rest of their team tries to guess.
- No verbal forms of communication – written or spoken – can be used to assist the group (grunting included).
- No numbers or internationally recognised symbols, like dollar signs, flags, the Red Cross, etc are permitted.

If you're familiar with the board

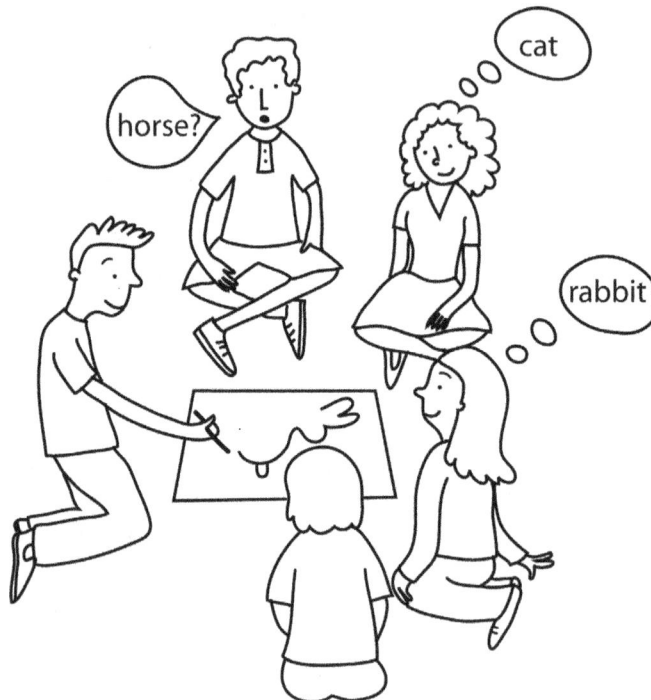

game, this version is a bit like playing a huge 'All Play' round. To start, ask one person from each group to approach you, and to creep in nice and close because you are about to whisper the first 'thing' they have to draw. Working from an already-prepared list (of say 40 – 50 things), whisper the first object in their shell-like – it could be a person, place, animal, action, thing, etc – check their understanding, and they're off!

Each 'artist' returns to their group, and, as quickly yet effectively as possible, tries to draw the 'thing.' When someone in their group correctly guesses its identity, another person from this team will race back to the front of the room to seek the next 'thing' to draw. Suggest to your group that keeping their voices down will prevent them from 'giving the answer away' to other groups.

At this point, you have to be quite organised. You only have one list (unless you share copies of it with other leaders to share the load of a very large group), so begin by asking the budding artist – who has just raced up to you – to tell you what was the last 'thing' drawn by his or her group. If you receive the correct answer (i.e., it's on your list), then whisper the next 'thing' on your list. If the answer is not correct, simply ask them to return to their group until they get it right. This way, groups can progress at their own speed.

You start with one person from each group, but beyond this, people will simply stream back to you in whatever order their groups have guessed the latest 'thing.' Stop when your list has run out, or you have been running for more than 30 minutes. A fun way to finish is to ask each group to gather their canvases and display them for the whole group to see.

Variations

- Create a list that reflects the significant people, things and events that have occurred during the course of your program or are relevant to the experiences of the group (in this way, the activity can act as a processing tool).

- Rather than draw, use charades or mime. That is, the 'artist' must use a series of physical gestures to communicate the message. As a further challenge, create a list of popular movies, TV shows or songs for this person to communicate.

- Rather than draw, use play dough. Each person will manipulate and mould the play dough to look like the 'thing.'

LEANING TOWER OF FEETZA

A creative way to use a bunch of shoes that really gets the brain ticking

AT A GLANCE

Small groups compete to build the tallest, free-standing structure they can, using only their shoes.

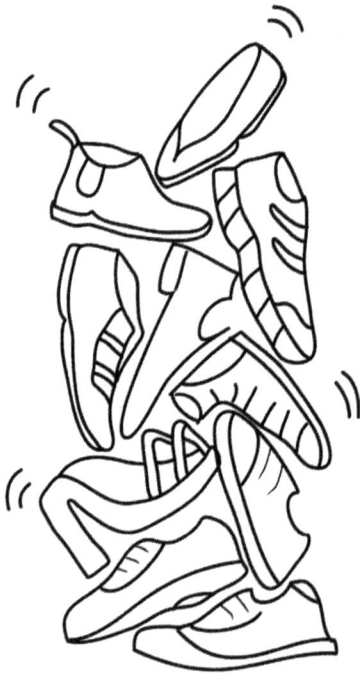

WHAT YOU NEED

A group wearing any type of footwear

10 – 15 mins

WHAT TO DO

The simplest activities are often the best.

Separate your gathering into small groups of any number – say 10 to 20 people – and ask them to sit together. Now, explain that their goal as a small group is to build the tallest free-standing structure they can, using only the riches of their shoes. Give them no longer than five minutes. Go!

Some groups will stretch the true meaning of what 'free-standing' means, but by my definition, it means that nothing – no seat, no hands, no walls, etc – can be used to keep the growing tower upright.

When time's up, ask for everyone to step away from their structures, and perform some form of measuring ritual to determine which tower is the tallest.

Variations

- Using feet only (shoes included), each small group will work together to form an unbroken chain of feet (touching each other, often end to end) from the floor to a point as high off the floor as possible. A safety note – it won't be long before someone realises that to get the 'tower' really high, you have to start lifting people off the ground, so that they can elevate their feet to the top of the growing tower. When this occurs, instruct the group to physically support these elevated people.

- As above, each person can only use one of their feet / shoes to form a part of the tower (requires a much larger group).

HUMAN MACHINES

A wonderfully inventive improvisation game for small groups

AT A GLANCE

Small groups of people work together, using their bodies to form a physical representation of a series of machines as they are announced by the leader.

WHAT YOU NEED

15 – 30 mins

WHAT TO DO

There's no magic number as to the size of your small groups with this one. Anything from 4 to 20 people is fine. The more people, the more complex your machine can be.

Having situated your small groups in different corners of your playing space, explain that you want every group to design and build their very own representation of a series of machines, which you will soon announce. Everyone in the group must be valuably involved, and the machine should demonstrate how it works with moving parts and functions like the real thing.

Some good machines to try are a Dishwasher, Washing Machine, Toilet, Motor Vehicle, CD Player and SLR Camera.

Give them two to four minutes to discuss how they will build their machine, and then ask each group one at a time to present their creations. Announce the next machine.

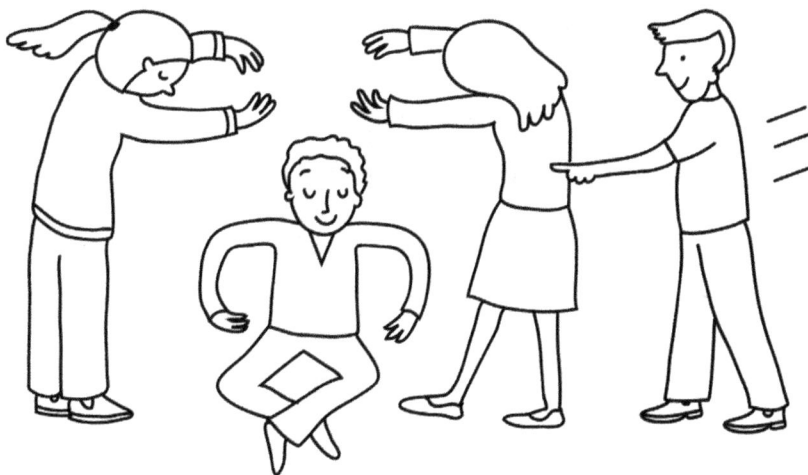

Variation

Announce a series of very simple machines and objects (table and chairs, a forest, a house, map of the world), but this time, allow no time for the group to think. They must immediately spring into action and improvise.

STICK AROUND

About as much fun as you can have with a roll of duct tape

AT A GLANCE

A small group attempts to use a roll of duct tape to stick one of their members to a wall.

WHAT YOU NEED

A wide, solid, non-painted wall
Roll of duct tape for each group
20 – 30 mins

WHAT TO DO

We all know that there is little that duct tape can't fix. Well, how about a person to a wall?

First up, you want to scope your venue for a suitable wall. You can immediately rule out any walls that have been painted, or those that are made of plaster. Use these, and there's a good chance this activity will do more than just damage your reputation. Rather, look for a wide, solid, unpainted cinderblock, concrete or brick wall. Timber can work, but it must be paint-free. And, if the wall is supporting a roof, it's probably strong enough.

Now, armed with a box of duct tape rolls, separate your multitude into random small groups of say six to eight people. Supply each group with a roll of duct tape, and explain in the simplest of terms that they each have 10 (to 15) minutes to suspend, hang or otherwise attach one of their group members to the wall.

Perhaps it's the thought of playing with duct tape, or maybe it's more about pinning one of their mates to a wall. But I am yet to see a group that

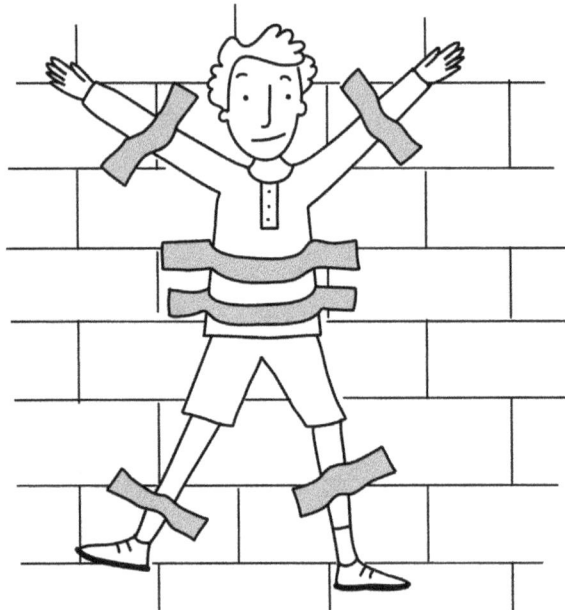

doesn't get that excited-little-boy look in their eyes when they hear about this challenge.

To complete the task, a group must be able to suspend one of their own for at least ten seconds, unassisted.

A few words about safety. The feet of the suspended should not be more than 60 cm (2') off the ground, and the application of tape should be preferably and carefully applied to clothing and not (hairy) skin.

Variations

- Consider any number of other awkward or heavy items to suspend on the wall.

- Using only a limited supply of duct tape, say 5 metres (17'), try hanging an object from the underside of a table, or the top of a door frame.

COLD SHOULDER

Perfect small group problem-solver for a hot day

AT A GLANCE
Small groups attempt to be the first to wear a t-shirt that has been frozen in a block of ice.

WHAT YOU NEED
A frozen t-shirt for each small group
10 – 15 mins

WHAT TO DO
The first thing you need to do is prepare the t-shirts. Grab a bunch of really old ones, because it is highly likely that they may not be worn again. For every small group, place one t-shirt into a small tub such as an ice-cream container, fill it with water and then stick it in your freezer overnight.

Next, remove the tubs, and present a mind-boggling array of frozen blocks of ice to your now-curious group. Explain that when you say "GO," each group will aim to (i) break open the block of ice to get at the t-shirt (which rests inside – ah, they didn't know!), and (ii) be the first small group to have someone wear the more than frost-bitten t-shirt.

Simple and as hard as that. I have seen everything from bashing the block against a concrete surface, to sitting it atop of a car's engine. Lots of crazy, frenetic pleasure.

Variation

Try socks for an easier challenge.

AUDIENCE FUN

After a period of high-energy, interactive, large group activity, it may be time for a change of pace. Perhaps your group needs to catch their breath, or you want to occupy some idle time, but you don't want to push everyone into 'doing' something.

This section presents a selection of some of the most successful, proven and funnest activities that passionately involve a small group of participants, which the rest of your group will adore as the 'audience.'

Or, put another way, if you need every person in your group to be actively 'doing' something, this section won't pay the bills. Rather, the focus here is to foster passive forms of participation, at a minimum.

So, these 'audience' style activities typically feature:

- An opportunity for one to six people to attract the 'focus' of their group
- Emphasis on fun, laughter and amusement
- Audience participation is optional, yet encouraged
- 15 to 60 minutes of play

Here are my favourites, presented in a sequence generally reflecting increasing levels of audience interaction and participant difficulty. Enjoy!

Minute Mysteries
The Story Game
Celebrity Head
Black Magic
The Psychiatrist
Charade Line
Taboo
Improv Games
In the Manner of the Word
B.F. Skinner
I Need A Shoelace
Paper Bag Pick-up

MINUTE MYSTERIES

A series of perplexing mysteries for your group to solve

AT A GLANCE

The brief facts of one or more 'mysteries' are presented to a group. Group members are invited to ask a series of 'Yes / No' questions to solve what happened in each case.

WHAT YOU NEED

List of 'mysteries'
10 – 30 mins

WHAT TO DO

You either love these little 'minute' mysteries, or you hate them – either way, it's often because the mystery takes much longer than a minute to solve!

These mysteries are a wonderful way to occupy idle moments because they take no time to set up, require no equipment and can be 'solved' on the run as well as sitting down. For example, I have often presented one or more mysteries to a group as we walk between two spots or journey in a vehicle. Or, in a residential setting, they have been presented over a meal.

This is the basic set-up. You gather your group, perhaps sit them down (it will often take longer than a minute!) and present the 'facts, the whole facts and nothing but the facts.' After they have digested the facts, invite your group to ask a series of questions that can be answered only with a "YES," "NO" or "IRRELEVANT" reply.

Here's one of the most classic minute mysteries to get you started:

"ROMEO AND JULIET ARE DEAD, LYING IN A PUDDLE OF WATER WITH BROKEN GLASS EVERYWHERE. HOW DID THEY DIE?"

Hmmmm? There are just so many lines of enquiry which may follow this information. However, it is critical that you only respond to 'Yes / No' questions. For example, do not answer "HOW OLD WERE THEY?" but "ARE THEY HUMAN?" is cool. Often times, a group will ask questions that are irrelevant or do not help the group to get closer to a solution. If this occurs, simply say "IRRELEVANT," and invite another question.

As the minutes tick by, your group will narrow their focus and finally arrive at the solution. It's frustrating, it's exciting and most of all it's fun. By the way, the answer to that second question above is "NO." The solution? Romeo and Juliet were fish, and their fish tank fell and crashed to the floor. Poor fishies.

Check out page 237 for more ready-made mysteries for you to pose.

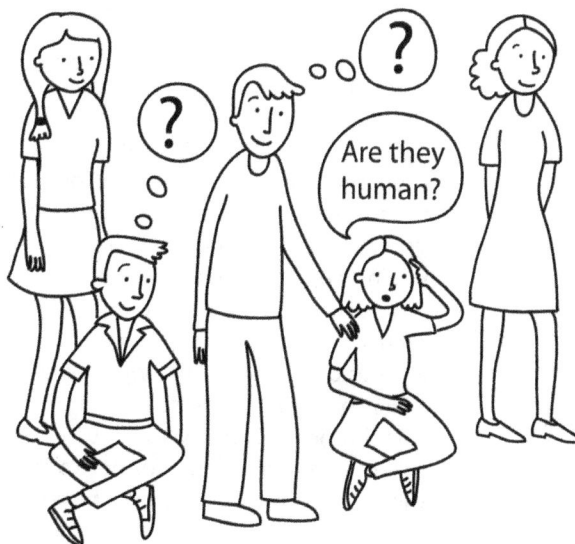

Variations

- Separate into small groups, and issue each group a unique mystery, or several of the same mysteries to solve.

- For the creatively-inspired, ask a small group to invent their own 'mystery' and challenge another group to solve it.

THE STORY GAME

A terribly fun way to tell a story

AT A GLANCE

An individual attempts to recreate a story developed by the rest of the group without their knowledge, by simply asking 'Yes / No' questions.

WHAT YOU NEED

10 – 20 minutes

WHAT TO DO

This game is so horrible, it's wonderful. Unlike many other games, there really is a trick to this one, and everyone knows about it except for one poor soul.

With everyone still bunched together, explain to your group that, in a moment, one person will leave the room, and while they are gone, the group will develop a short story that everyone needs to remember. The task for the individual who will volunteer to go first, is to recreate the story with a beginning, a middle and an end. And this person can only create the elements of the story by asking the group a series of questions that will garner "YES" or "NO" answers.

At this point, identify your 'story teller,' and then ask him or her to leave the space. Now, the thing we haven't said is that there is no story, but the 'story-teller' doesn't know this. Explain that all your group has to do is agree on two 'things' that will appear in the story which the 'story-teller' will (in effect) make up. Also, one of these things must end with a vowel, and the other end with a consonant. For purposes of illustration, let's say the two things are 'koala' and 'train.'

Now, explain that when the story teller asks a question, any time it (the sentence) ends with a consonant, the answer is "YES" and when it ends with a vowel, the answer is "NO." Simple and as tricky as that!

So, let the story begin. The story teller re-enters the space, and is told that to assist him or her in the creation of the story, there are two things that are featured – in this case – a koala and a train. The story teller launches into their first question, and with confidence that will fool the story teller into thinking that the group is very clear about their story, will receive an emphatic "YES" to every consonant-ending question and a resounding "NO" on a vowel-ending question.

Oh, it's so cruel, but really it's not – because, the delight that is exhibited on a story teller's face when he or she concocts the most absurd element to a story, and yet the group answers with a "YES" is priceless. 'I-am-so-good-at-this' will be written all over his or her face. Of course, there are occasions when the facts don't seem to make sense, when a question is answered one way (because it ended in a vowel the first time), but is answered differently the next time (because it ended in a consonant). It's all part of the thrill of the chase.

As facilitator, be sure to keep the story moving, by encouraging the story teller to keep going over the facts of the story as they know it. Look for a beginning, a middle and an end. At some point, when it appears the story has reached a conclusion, support ample praise for a job well done. And then reveal the true story – there really was no story!

Variation

Invite two or more people to become the story tellers.

CELEBRITY HEAD

A game in which the audience knows you better than you do

AT A GLANCE

With the name of a 'celebrity' stuck to their foreheads, four people will attempt to identify who the celebrity is by asking an audience a limited number of 'Yes / No' questions about this person.

WHAT YOU NEED
  Set of 'celebrity' name-tags
  Sticky tape
  15 – 30 mins

WHAT TO DO

The set-up for this exercise is very similar to that of Who Am I? Rather than repeat myself, may I suggest you read the initial set-up of this activity on page 56, and then come on back.

OK, I can safely assume you have a set of index cards with the names of well-known, celebrity type people written on them. Gather your group, and invite three or four volunteers to become 'celebrities.' They take their seat at the

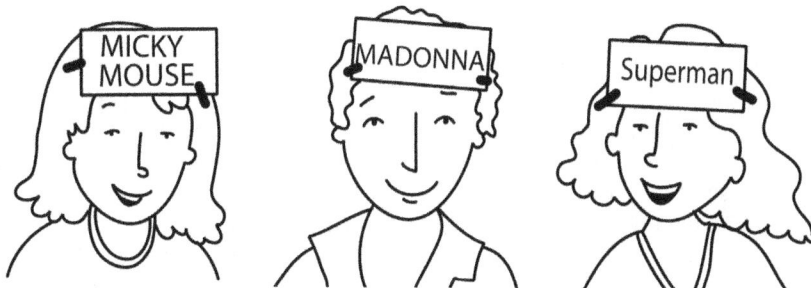

front of your playing space, and you stick an index card on each of their foreheads. As long as the person to whom the index card belongs cannot see their celebrity status, anyone can view the card, celebrity or otherwise.

Next, explain that the mission for each 'celebrity' is to identify 'who they are' by asking the rest of their group (the audience) as few 'Yes / No' questions as possible. That is, a celebrity is only permitted to ask a question that can be answered "YES" or "NO."

It works like this. A celebrity will ask the first question, and upon receiving the group's reply, the next celebrity in line will ask their question, and so on.

Challenge the celebrities to identify who they are within ten (or so) questions. Once a celebrity has guessed their identity, ask for someone from the audience to swap spots with them. Or, wait until all celebrities have been identified before introducing a new set of people.

The tension is much greater than in Who Am I? because there are a whole lot more people watching this amusing identity crisis.

Note: If you have trouble sticking the index cards onto people's foreheads, introduce a number of hats for the celebrities to wear, onto which you stick their identity.

Variation

Allow the 'celebrity' to continue asking questions until they receive a "NO" from the group, at which point, the next celebrity may ask their question.

BLACK MAGIC

Ideal activity to fill a few idle minutes around the camp-fire

AT A GLANCE

One person, acting as a 'mind reader,' correctly identifies a series of objects that his or her group has secretly nominated before he or she enters the room.

WHAT YOU NEED

20 – 30 mins

WHAT TO DO

This exercise can be so much fun and will fill many idle minutes of your program. I'll present the most basic version, and then a few variations of the 'trick.'

Gather your group and seat them comfortably – they could be there for a while. Announce that you would like one person – a colleague, or one of your group members – to leave the area so that they cannot see or hear what is about to transpire. Upon their departure, explain that you would like the group to nominate some object (that everyone can see) for this volunteer to identify when they return. Let's say they pick my guitar. Cool.

The volunteer returns – let's call him or her the 'mind reader.' The 'mind reader's' task is to correctly identify the object that the group has just picked. Now, what the group does not know is the 'trick.' You see, in advance of the group assembling, you and this volunteer have discussed what the 'trick' is going to be. You are limited only by your imagination, but for now, I'll use the 'object-suggested-directly-after-a-black-object' trick.

Here's how it works. You welcome the 'mind-reader' back into the group, and announce that an object has been chosen, and explain that you will suggest a particular item, and he or she will confirm or deny if this is it. So, I might say, "IS IT THIS CHAIR?," and the mind-reader shakes his or her head. "IS IT THE PLATE?" and again he or she shakes a No. "IS IT THE SHOE?," again negative. But, the Mind-Reader notes that the shoe is black, so this telegraphs to him or her that the next object will be 'it.' Pointing next at the chosen object, I say "IS IT MY GUITAR?" and the Mind-Reader says "YES!" Voila! Your group sits there amazed with 'How-did-they-do-that?' written all over their faces.

Repeat this process over and over. After several rounds, some folks will start to catch on. If so, test their new-found magical powers, and invite them to become a 'mind-reader' too. However, if you are like me, and hate being left in the dark for too long, you may gradually provide more and more clues to the group (so that they may catch on to the trick) until at the very end, you explicitly describe what's happening.

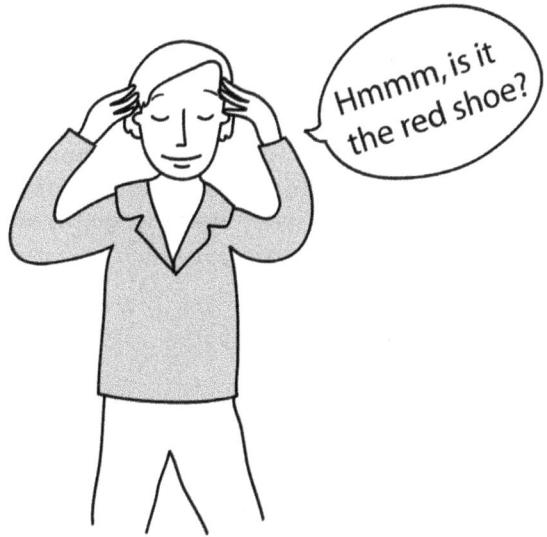

Perhaps a trick too easy to pick? Maybe, so try one of these...

Variations

- The first letter of the first word the 'leader' speaks to the 'mind-reader' (as they re-enter the space) will inform the 'mind-reader' that the object starts with this letter. For example, I may say "GREAT, YOU'RE BACK, I WANT YOU.... " blah blah blah, if the object was my guitar.

- Assemble a collection of five to ten random items in front of your group. Situated in a line, secretly label them A, B, C, D, etc. The group secretly picks one of these items. Inform the 'mind reader' that the first letter of the first word you use when they return to the space is the item. For example, if the chosen item is secretly labelled 'F' (which happens to be a book), I might say, "FORGET YOUR MAGIC, IT WON'T WORK..."

THE PSYCHIATRIST

A clever 'what's-the-key' exercise that may drive you crazy

AT A GLANCE

One person asks a group of people a series of questions in an attempt to identify the secret 'rule' that guides all of their responses.

WHAT YOU NEED

15 – 30 mins

WHAT TO DO

Standard set-up. You need one person to leave the room, so that they don't hear what you will discuss with the rest of the group. However, before they leave, describe what happens.

Explain that after the volunteer (the 'psychiatrist') leaves the space, the rest of your group will decide on one specific rule to follow when answering all of the 'psychiatrist's' questions. For example:

- Answer all questions in five words.
- Begin all sentences with a vowel.
- Begin all sentences with the last letter of the question.
- Subtly clear one's throat just before speaking.

- Answer without blinking.

Guide your group to not make the rule too difficult, lest the volunteer really need to seek professional help.

So, the group agrees on a rule, the 'psychiatrist' re-enters the space, sits down in front of his or her 'patients,' and starts asking a series of questions. Simple stuff like, "HARRY, DID YOU WALK TO SCHOOL?" and "HOW ARE YOU, BRUCE?" The 'psychiatrist' continues to ask questions – one question of one person at a time – until they finally discover the rule.

If several minutes have passed, or you note that the 'psychiatrist' is losing enthusiasm, invite your group to start giving a few clues, i.e., by making the 'rule' more obvious. Remember, it's not a test, it's supposed to be fun. If a group watches one of their own 'suffer' for too long, you can bet no one will want to go next.

Note: This activity works with all group sizes. Everyone simply needs to be able to hear the psychiatrist reach a diagnosis.

Variations

- Try it with two or three 'psychiatrists' working together as a team.
- Mix this exercise with In The Manner of the Word on page 203. The 'psychiatrist' has to identify the adverb chosen by the group from the manner in which they answer their questions.

CHARADE LINE

Chinese whispers in the form of a mime

AT A GLANCE

Five people are invited, one person at a time, to watch a short story being mimed to them, with the objective of passing the story along to the next person in line.

WHAT YOU NEED

20 – 30 minutes

WHAT TO DO

Invite five people from your group to join you in the centre of the 'performance area.' Ask these folks to form a straight line facing away from you so that everyone is facing the back of the person in front of them. Next, tap the shoulder of the person closest to you, and ask that person only to turn around and face you.

Their task is to observe closely everything that you (as story teller) are about to 'perform,' because very shortly, they will have to replicate this story exactly as they see it. The 'story teller' cannot speak or use any verbal communication whatsoever, just simply mime their story. Much like a pantomime, stories that involve lots of movement, have a beginning, a middle and an end, and last about 30 seconds work best.

Can't think of a story? No worries. Look at page 238 for a series of stories that I've already road-tested for you.

So, other than the 'audience,' only the person you have tapped will have been party to your story. You sit down, and explain that this person now taps the next person in line, and repeats

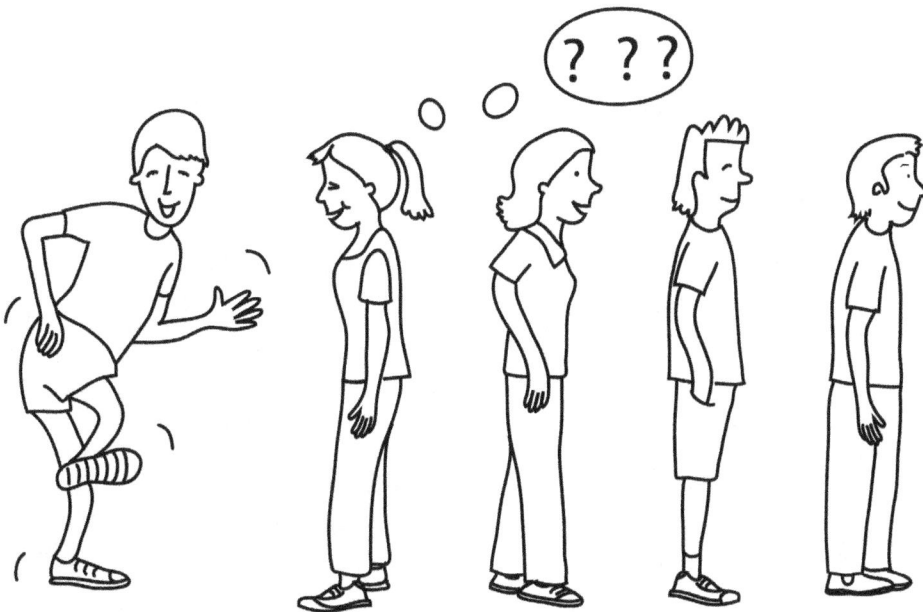

the story exactly as they remember it, which on average is about 60% of what actually transpired, and 40% that never did. This process continues all the way down the line. As you can imagine, much like Chinese Whispers, the story is bound to get warped along the way.

During the re-telling of the story, the audience is permitted to laugh (a lot), but never indicate or say anything to suggest that the story is 'wrong.' They should simply sit back and enjoy. Some of the most painful laughing fits I have ever experienced have occurred as a result of this activity.

Once the last person observes the story re-told for the fifth time (in the eyes of the audience), most of the fun will have been had. But, for a few more laughs, it's worthwhile asking each person, starting from this very last person and working back up to the start of the line, to re-tell the story as they 'saw' it happen.

The game completes with the person who first introduced the story performing it again, mostly for the benefit of those who stood in line and had their backs turned away at the time it was first shown.

Variation

Invite two people to mime a story to another pair, the first in a line of I've-got-my-back-to-you pairs. You can provide some thinking time for the initial story tellers to develop their story. Or, to be held totally in suspense, allow the process to be improvised, so the initial story is created by the first story tellers spontaneously.

TABOO

A fast-paced, frenetic word game that will get your group thinking

AT A GLANCE

Within a set time limit, one person stands in front of a list of words – which he or she cannot see – and considers the verbal clues of his or her team – who can see the list – to correctly identify as many of the words as possible.

WHAT YOU NEED
List of 'objects' or 'things' (optional)
Large sheets of paper
Marker pens
Sticky tape
30 – 45 mins

WHAT TO DO

This is a classic re-working of the popular board game 'Taboo,' but easier and loads more fun with a larger group assisting the poor sod out front.

Here's the basic set-up. Pin a large sheet of paper (flip-chart paper is ideal) on a wall or easel-type thing. Ask one person to volunteer to stand in front of the paper, with his or her back to the paper, facing the group. Either guided by a list you have prepared in advance, or simply making them up on the spot, write four objects or things in large letters on the paper. For example, FILING

CABINET, BBQ, THERMOMETER, SPAIN, etc. Naturally, the group can see this list, but the volunteer cannot.

You are now good to go. The goal is for the group to call out a series of clues to their unknowing team-mate to help him or her guess what all four things are that are written on the list – all in 60 seconds. The words can be worked in any order; however, to keep it fair and fun, there are a set of 'rules' that need to be followed:

- No part of a thing or object can be mentioned; for example if the object is 'PAINT BRUSH,' the group cannot say "PAINT" or "BRUSH" as separate words
- No hand gestures or motions – only verbal communication
- No 'sounds-like' or rhyming words

If a 'rule' is broken, the word that was guessed as a result is not counted. How the group conducts itself as it tries to communicate is totally up to the group. In the beginning, there is often a lot of shouting over the top of one another, before the group catches on to how it can be more effective. Some valuable teachable moments here that you may choose to debrief later, perhaps?

Anyway, with each 60-second period, produce a new set of words and a new volunteer to do the guessing. Challenge the group to correctly identify as many words as possible within, say, 30 minutes.

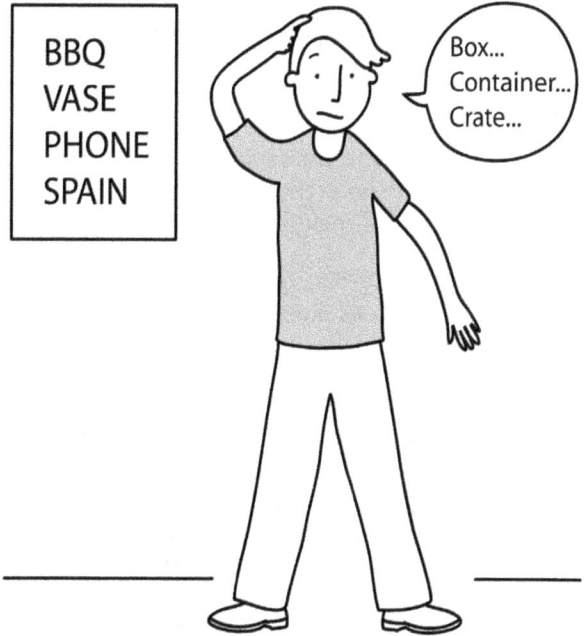

BBQ
VASE
PHONE
SPAIN

Box...
Container...
Crate...

Variation

With large numbers, separate your group into two or three teams. Provide a unique set of words for each group, and award points to each correctly-guessed word. The team with the highest number of points at the end of several rounds wins.

IMPROV GAMES

A series of activities that rely on your group's impulsive creativity

AT A GLANCE

One or more people take on the challenge to create and play out a 'story' with no preparation, to entertain the rest of their group.

WHAT YOU NEED

15 – 45 mins

WHAT TO DO

There are just so many fantastic improvisational games out there, I couldn't possibly list them all (that's why other people have chosen to write books about them). Nevertheless, I will share a few of my favourites and hopefully inspire you to incorporate a few improv activities into your program.

You see, improv is 'adventure' in its purest form – unanticipated outcomes. So if you're looking for something that will excite, challenge and inspire your group to think creatively and work together, then improv has it going on!

The games that follow are a form of 'theatre' in which the players 'think on their feet' to perform spontaneously. The quality of the performance rarely matters – it's all about being creative, moving the story-line forward and working with others. On some occasions, you will ask your group (the audience) to offer the players a few suggestions to guide their performance as they create dialogue, setting, and the plot.

One Word At A Time

Ask four or five people to sit or stand in front of the group. Upon receiving a suggestion for a 'place' (i.e., where the characters in the story are situated), the volunteers will tell a story one word at a time. For example, Fred says "WHEN," then Daisy says "THE," and Jerry follows with "CAT" and so on, each word adding to and moving the story forward. When the last person in line says their word, the story continues from the first person again.

New Identity

Place any item (frisbee, piece of fabric, a fork, etc) in front of your group. Ask for one person at a time to run to the front, pick up the item and imagine it to be something it obviously isn't. For example, someone may place the frisbee on the ground, stand on it and then pretend that it is a flying saucer they are riding. As soon as the item's 'identity' is established, a new person must race to the front and invent a new identity. The quicker the change-over and inventing, the better.

What Are You Doing?

One person starts at the front doing any recognisable movement, such as directing traffic, riding a horse or running a race. Within seconds, another person will tap this person on the shoulder, and ask "WHAT ARE YOU DOING?" at which point the first person must immediately reply with a suggestion of some other action (that they are in fact not doing). This second person must immediately perform this new action. For example, Penny starts by watering her pot plants, and then upon Yvonne's approach, Penny replies that she is riding an elephant.

Yvonne departs the stage and Penny immediately makes like riding an elephant.

Diminishing Scene

Invite four people to move into the performance space. Ask your group to offer three things, a 'place,' an 'object' and a 'celebrity.' The object for the volunteers is to perform a short one-minute story that incorporates all three things. Ideally, the story should have a beginning, a middle and an end. Once performed, the same four people repeat the story, but in half the time, i.e., 30 seconds. And then a third time in 15 seconds and finally, in 7.5 seconds.

Expert Interview

Ask a confident person to sit in a chair facing the rest of their group to pose as an 'international expert.' The subject of this person's expertise will be suggested by the group. For example, from all of the suggestions, you choose 'Rare African Dung Beetle.' One at a time, you invite a volunteer to approach the 'expert' and ask an important question. The expert immediately invents a convincing reply.

Variation

Enter "improvisational games" into an internet search engine, and prepare to be dazzled with more ideas than you can imagine.

IN THE MANNER OF THE WORD

An intriguing problem-solving activity that will improve your vocabulary

AT A GLANCE

A small group of people act in the manner of an adverb they have chosen corresponding to a series of 'situations' suggested by their audience.

WHAT YOU NEED

List of adverbs (optional)
20 – 30 mins

WHAT TO DO

I warn you now – this exercise can be a riot.

You need at least one volunteer to make this activity happen, but the more the merrier. So, if you ask for a volunteer and you get five hands, take them all.

Ask these volunteers to assemble at the front of the room or performance space and explain that they (as a group) need to secretly think of one adverb, you know, a word that ends with '-ly.' Any adverb is kosher, but encourage them to think of a fun adverb such as slowly, nervously, or eagerly.

OK, with these folks standing out in front, you are ready to go. You now ask the rest of the group – the audience, so to speak – to offer a series of 'situations' for the volunteers to

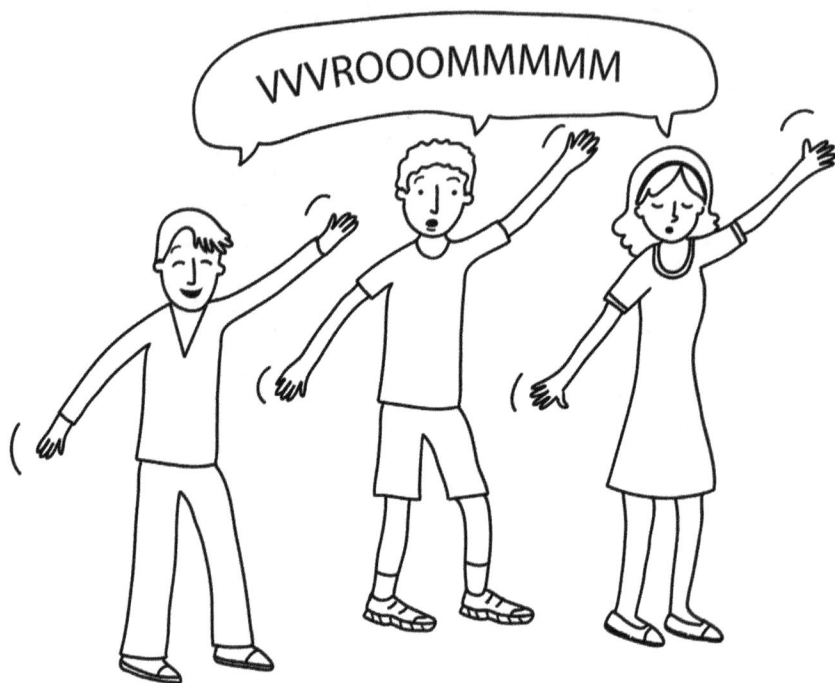

perform, one at a time. For example, the situation could be 'brushing your teeth,' or 'flying a plane.' Upon each suggestion, the volunteers perform the situation in the manner of the adverb they have chosen. The goal is for the audience to correctly guess the adverb as quickly as possible.

If, after playing a particular situation for ten or more seconds, the audience has not correctly identified the adverb, ask your group to offer another situation. The situations and acts continue until the adverb is guessed. If several minutes pass, feel free to ask the performers to offer a few clues.

Sometimes, I have a list of adverbs up my sleeve just in case the group runs out of ideas. See page 238 for a list of adverbs that are fun to act out.

Variations

- As above, but the players acting out the adverbs can only mime their performance.

- One or more volunteers leave the room. The rest of the group decides which adverb they will perform. The volunteers return to the playing space, and describe a series of 'situations' for the whole group to perform. Works best if the volunteers stand in the middle of the action.

B.F. SKINNER

A game that celebrates the discovery of specific kinds of human movements

AT A GLANCE

Two people work together in front of an appreciative audience to discover – through trial and error – an exact position and / or movement that the rest of the group had 'created' before the pair entered the space.

WHAT YOU NEED

20 – 30 minutes

WHAT TO DO

In a moment, you will ask for two volunteers to leave the space, so that the rest of the group can work on a problem. There are no tricks up your sleeve, but you are well advised to explain everything to everyone before this pair departs.

The object for the two volunteers is to correctly demonstrate the exact position and / or movement of two people, as identified secretly by the rest of the group. For example, while the pair is absent from the space, the rest of the group will invite two others to display what the 'desired position' looks like – perhaps one person lays with their back on the ground and their legs held up in the air by their partner. It's very

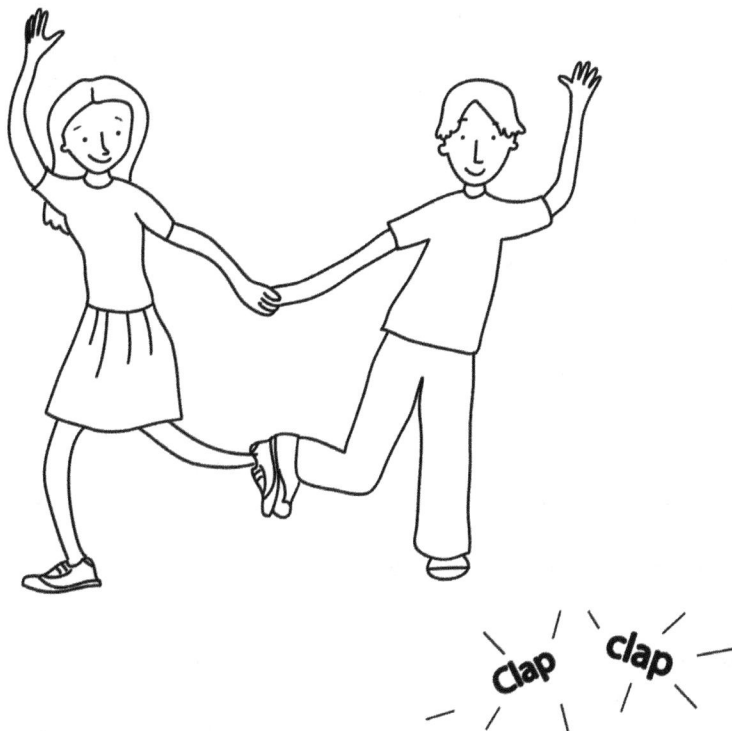

important that everyone has a clear idea about what they want the unknowing pair to achieve.

When everyone is ready, invite the pair to enter the 'performance area,' and work together by means of trial and error to achieve the desired position and / or movements. The group cannot speak to the pair, nor can they answer any questions. The only feedback the pair will receive from the group is their applause. When the pair 'do' something that resembles one or more parts of the desired positions – for example, one of them suddenly lies on the ground – the group will increase the pace of their applause. It's a lot like the 'getting warmer' game you played at school. The closer the pair gets to the exact position, the warmer and more joyous the applause.

Most pairs will 'get it' within five minutes. Beyond this, if there is a risk the pair will simply throw in the towel, feel free to offer a few hints such as what part of their bodies they could focus on moving. If the clapping is subdued, encourage the pair to do anything that is different from what they have been doing.

As facilitator, err on the side of 'structural ease' when guiding your group to create the desired position. If it's too complex, with too many refined positions, the pair may never 'get it,' and that's no fun for anybody. Keep it simple.

Expect some classic moments of humour and side-splitting laughter from the audience as the unknowing pair struggle to find the 'answer.' And be sure that when they do, the group offers their most frenzied applause.

Oh, and by the way. B.F. Skinner was well known for his study of human behaviour and movement. Does the name of the game make sense now?

Variation

Involve three or four people to create a position in which every person is physically connected in some way to the others.

I NEED A SHOELACE

A treasure hunt with a difference

AT A GLANCE

Two or more groups compete to be the fastest to produce a series of nominated objects or things that a 'leader' randomly requests.

WHAT YOU NEED
List of 'things'
15 – 30 mins

WHAT TO DO

Think of this as a kind of urgent treasure hunt. Split your group into two, three or four teams, and ask each team to find a spot to sit together that is roughly an equal distance from you (so no team feels disadvantaged).

Explain that you will soon announce a series of random, yet generally common

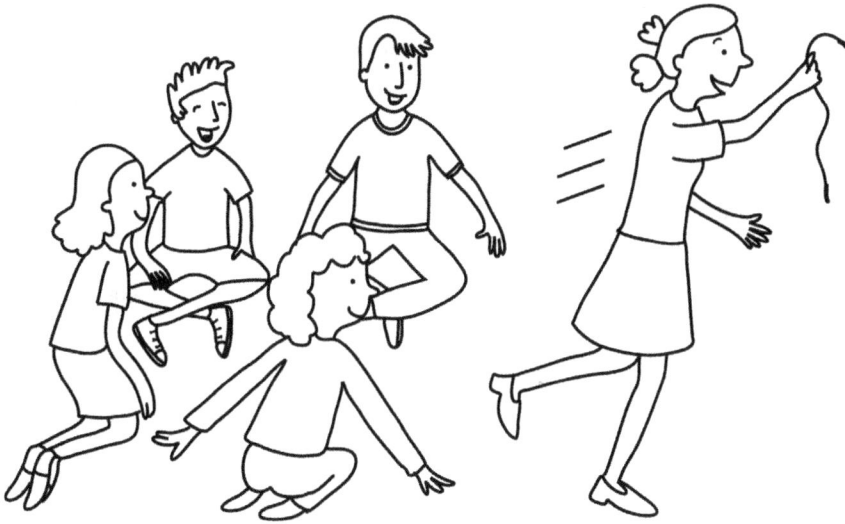

objects or things, and the first group to present these things to you will win that round. Pretty basic.

Of course, there is no limit (other than appropriateness) to what you could demand of your group. To get you started, this list of 'things' seems to work pretty well:

Shoelace
Driver's License
8 shoes tied together
Flower
Chewed gum

Someone with food in their teeth
Sock with a hole in it
3 belts hooked together
Stub of a movie ticket
Coin made in 1980
Comb

To avoid the inevitable crush of groups rushing at you from time to time, allow only one person from each team to approach you. Also, I often place a rubber spot (or chalk circle) for each team at least 2 metres (7') in front of me to represent their 'show-and-tell' area.

Variation

Adding a more physical element to this exercise, take a look at Be Prepared on page 213. The 'treasure' in this instance is a series of (often physical) tasks that need to be accomplished, for example, "FORM A LINE AND LEAP-FROG EVERYONE IN YOUR GROUP."

PAPER BAG PICK-UP

A simple game-turned-stunt that will astound you

AT A GLANCE

A group, one person at a time, will attempt to lift a slowly-diminishing paper bag off the floor using their mouth, with only their feet ever touching the ground.

WHAT YOU NEED

One regular grocery paper bag

15 – 30 mins

WHAT TO DO

Be careful with this one, and I don't just mean its physicality. It is totally intoxicating too.

Find a moment when your group is just sitting around, pretty much idle. Pull out a paper bag – you know, the kind that supermarkets fill with groceries – and puff it open so that it sits upright and stiff in the midst of your group. If you didn't have it before, you will now have their full attention.

Announce that anyone may volunteer to pick up the paper bag. Yet, in order to 'officially' pick it up, explain that a person must use only their mouth to grab the bag, and they are not permitted to have anything other than their feet touch the ground during the process. That is, if during an attempt someone should fall forward or use their hands (or any other part of their anatomy) to brace themselves, this attempt will be deemed unofficial – as governed by the Official Paper Bag Pick-up Commission, of course!

At this point, you normally get a few takers. Suggest that these folk form a circle, and that each person take a turn to pick up the bag. Oh, but just one more thing. After each successful round, a volunteer is invited to tear a portion off the walls of the bag. So, if the bag ordinarily stands 40 cm tall (16"), someone may choose to rip off the top 10 cm (4") making the bag now stand only 30 cm (12") off the ground. Hmmm.

So, the process continues to rotate around the circle, and with each lap, the 'pick-up' gets a little harder as a

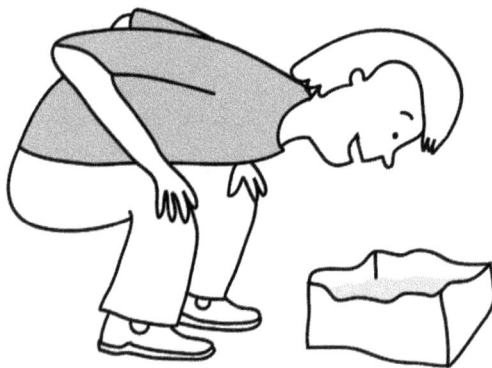

participant (who is still eligible) tears a ribbon of paper off the top of the ever-diminishing walls. Ultimately, believe it or not, the bag is always reduced to its base – that's right, it lies completely flat on the floor, naked of its walls!!

Using a paper bag is wise, because it leaves wet spot warnings for the players to work around (another reason why we rip off the top). By the way, official rules dictate that fully standing with the bag in one's mouth constitutes a 'pick-up,' and if a person does not officially lift the bag after three consecutive attempts (at the same height) they are eliminated.

Variation

Sorry, I haven't been able to invent a variation for this one. I'm still receiving physio from my last attempt!

MAJOR EVENTS

The activities described in this final section will easily fill an hour or two of your program. Think a little preparation, a nice open space, and a few easy-to-get-a-hold-of resources. Then add a lot of people, and you're ready to go.

Major events can be distinguished from all other activities because they typically feature:

- Activity that will occupy and involve a whole group for 1 to 2 hours
- A focus on lots of fun and interaction
- Intense preparation, staff and equipment needs.

Grouping activities of a similar format together, I present my favourite programmed group events.

Balloon-Arama
Be Prepared
Around The World
BlueStarOpoly
Mastermind Relay
The Great Egg Drop
Team Scrabble
Family Feud
Name That Tune
Scavenger Hunt
Treasure Hunt
City Search

BALLOON-ARAMA

Show me a bag of balloons, and I'll show you a bag full of fun

AT A GLANCE

A medley of fun, interactive 'balloon' activities that begin simply and become progressively more 'team' oriented.

WHAT YOU NEED

Loads of balloons

1 – 2 hours

WHAT TO DO

Every one of the activities I am about to describe can be presented in its own right. However, here are just eight ideas that will easily fill an hour or two, presented in a 'worked-many-times-before' sequence.

Brackwfffff

Everyone holds an inflated, but un-tied balloon in their hands, standing behind a line at one end of a hall or playing field. One at a time, each person lets go of their balloon to let it splutter and 'horsey' as far away from the line as possible. Have several attempts, the balloon reaching the furthest distance wins.

Balloon Orchestra

Everyone inflates their balloon as large as is reasonable, ties them off and assembles in a semi-circle formation facing you, the 'conductor.' You divide your assembly into four or five smaller groups, each representing a unique section of the orchestra which is asked to make a unique sound with their balloons. For example, one section rubs their balloons, another may pull on the neck of the balloon and let it go, while a third group may tap their balloons with their fingers. Instruct each section to do a quick sound test, and then raise your baton to command a royal philharmonic performance. Bring each section in individually, raise their volume, then soften them, etc, etc, finally building to a crescendo (don't pop them yet!) and stop! Ahhh, silence.

Boop

Separate into pairs. Place one balloon safely off to the side, and ask each duo to hold hands to form a circle. With the other balloon, explain that you will soon announce a part of the human anatomy which the pairs will use exclusively to keep the balloon off the ground. Try hands, then knees, heads, noses, shoulders, chests, feet, etc. Invite each pair to swap balloons with another pair mid-air. After much exercise, ask each partnership to stop and hold the balloon lightly between their co-joined hands. To finish, no touching is permitted to keep the balloon off the ground – the partners can only use their breath to keep the balloon aloft. Puff, puff, puff. Most people end up on the ground as a result.

Star Wars

Evenly distribute your group members throughout a wide, open area. Distribute one balloon to each person. Invite people to gently hit their balloons to keep them aloft. Boop, boop, boop. Then ask them to swap balloons with another person mid-air, aiming to keep all balloons off the ground at all times. Then, in a drastic scene change, invite each person to purposefully hit hips, etc. Their object is to rotate the balloon all the way up and down one of their bodies without using their limbs to assist its journey. A wild challenge. Next, have the balloon start on their tummies, and move the balloon down one person's body, under their legs, up their back and over the shoulder to return to their tummy. Even wilder.

Balloon Trolleys

New partners, one person facing the back of the other places one or two balloons between their bodies. Ask each pair to move about the area without losing their balloon(s). Ideally, they should not use their limbs to keep their balloons in situ. Challenge them to move rapidly, turn corners, go under obstacles, etc. Then, two pairs join, to form a balloon trolley of four people, a balloon (or two) between the back and tummy of each person. Again, move about the area. Next, a quad joins a quad, and finally two octuplets join to form a trolley of sixteen people. Provide a minute or so of practice, then assemble each 'team' behind a line, and race them from one end of the space to the other. The first team to return with all (or most) of their balloons wins.

Finally, the dilemma at the end of all this activity is to know what to do with all of the balloons. Here are two of my all-time crowd favourites.

Fire In The Hole

Separate into pairs. One partner places their balloon onto their belly, and invites his or her partner to press their belly against the balloon from the other side. Then, extending their arms around the other's back, each person

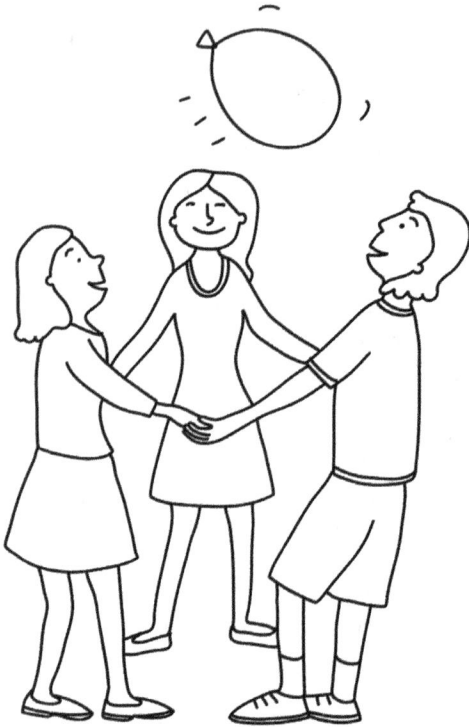

their balloon into the path of another, causing its owner a brief moment of 'lost control.' A chaotic scene, but fun nonetheless. If you wish, the owners of any balloons that drop to the ground are eliminated. Otherwise, continue to introduce new instructions, such as "ONLY HIT ANOTHER BALLOON OF THE SAME COLOUR," or "MOVE TO THE OTHER SIDE OF THE AREA USING YOUR NON-DOMINANT HAND." If the colour distribution is relatively even, announce that the team with the most balloons aloft at the end (or in two minutes) wins.

Up & Down

Each person finds a partner. Using just one of their balloons, they place it gently between any two parts of their bodies, such as their tummies, backs, pulls their partner closer to themselves, thereby exerting extreme pressure on the balloon until it pops! Repeat with next balloon.

Stress Balloon

Separate into pairs. Standing 1 metre (3') apart, partners face one another holding their balloons in their own two hands so that a balloon sits just in front of each person's chest. Wide-eyed and courageous, each person will apply mounting pressure to their balloon, maintaining eye contact with each other until either their balloon pops, or they turn defeated to look away! A real test, of nerves you could say.

Variation

What, you need more? OK, tie a balloon to the ankle of each person, ideally with a string that allows the balloon to drift a slight distance from the foot (to avoid stamping thereon). On "GO," each person aims to eliminate other people by stepping on and bursting their balloons, while preventing others from doing the same to their own. A real energiser.

BE PREPARED

A raucous medley of spontaneous small group activity and fun

AT A GLANCE

Sitting in front of a large number of sealed envelopes – each with a unique answer written on them – teams compete to be the first to accomplish the zany task that is revealed inside the envelope that corresponds with the leader's question.

WHAT YOU NEED

Many sheets of paper
List of zany activities
Box of envelopes
Set of questions, with answers
Various props, as determined by your activities
1 hour

WHAT TO DO

Warning, this one takes some time to prepare, but it's worth every minute.

There are three primary tasks:

1. Develop a list of 15 to 20 questions, with answers.
2. Write these answers onto the front of an envelope, one set of envelopes for every 'team.'
3. Develop a set of 15 to 20 zany activities or tasks (one per question) for your teams to accomplish.

To get you started and stir your creative juices, I have listed a ton of activity and task ideas on page 239. Here are three examples to illustrate:

"SHAKE THE HANDS OF AT LEAST THREE PEOPLE IN A NEIGHBOURING GROUP."
"EVERYONE SWAP A PIECE OF OUTER CLOTHING WITH SOMEONE ELSE IN YOUR GROUP, AND WEAR IT."

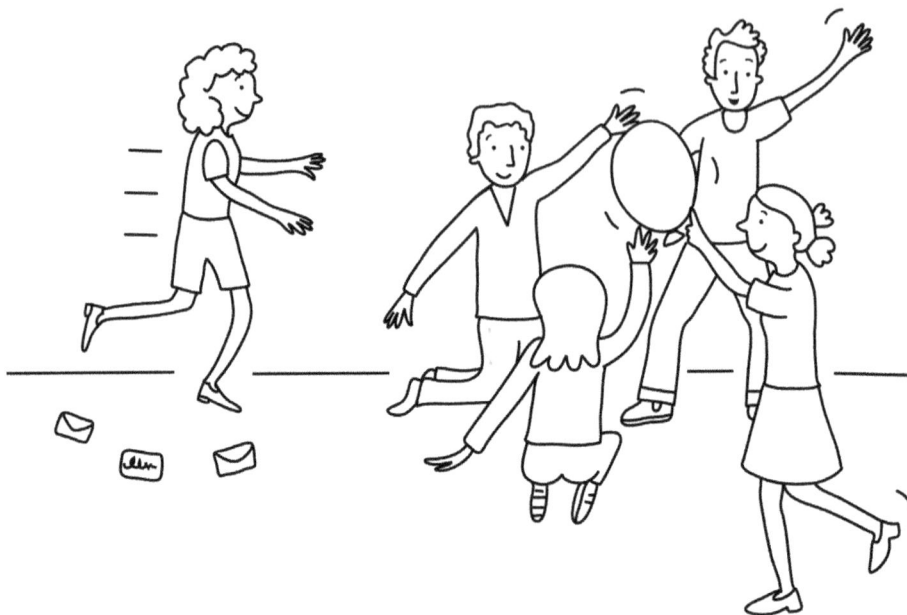

"INFLATE A BALLOON AND HAVE EVERYONE IN YOUR GROUP TOUCH THE BALLOON, WITHOUT TOUCHING ANYONE ELSE IN THE GROUP."

As for your questions, they can be as relevant or trivial as you want them to be. Looking back, I have asked everything from silly questions pertinent to the group I was working with, to a set of mathematical equations. The key is that your list of questions will produce an equal number of unique answers. That is, no two questions could be linked to the same answer.

Now, armed with your equal number of questions, answers and zany activities, you can prepare the envelopes. Your goal, to create a set of envelopes for every group that is identical, i.e., each envelope labelled with a particular answer will have the identical activity written on a small piece of paper inside of it. It's a tedious task, but very important to get right. Seal the envelopes to prevent sneaky preparedness.

Finally, to the play. Separate your group into small 'teams,' and spread them evenly throughout your playing area. Ask the team members to sit in a circle, and in the middle, fan out their set of envelopes, answers facing up. Next, you explain that you will ask a series of questions, and each team's goal is to identify the correct answer, open the corresponding envelope and perform the activity or task that is written on the paper inside. Often the measure of success is to identify which team accomplished the task first, but sometimes, it is the quality of the result that is assessed. Because no one knows the questions in advance, everyone has to be prepared for anything!

I tend to award nominal points to the team that 'wins' each round, accumulating team scores at the end, but it's not about the points, is it? To be honest, I can rarely tell which team is actually the first to accomplish a task – it's all about enjoying a serious bout of spontaneous fun!

Don't forget, see page 239 to view a set of ready-made activities and tasks.

Variation

Use the format of this exercise to test your group's knowledge about a certain topic, for example, the times table (multiplication).

AROUND THE WORLD

Excellent circuit-based program for keeping large groups of people active, and having fun, for a long time

AT A GLANCE
Groups of people rotate between a series of zany team activities with an emphasis on interaction and having fun.

WHAT YOU NEED
Varies depending on the activities you choose

A map of the 'world' for each team, to help guide them around the course (optional)

1 to 2 hours

WHAT TO DO
Before we get to the mechanics of the program, you need to picture this. Imagine a series of activities – one after another – that can take 10 to 15 minutes for a small group to complete, located at various 'stations' throughout your venue. One small group or 'team' is located at a particular activity at any point in time, and will rotate through-out the various stations (referred to as countries of the world) moving between the stations in a prescribed sequence at periodic intervals during the course of the program. Phew, did you get that?

Ideally, you will have access to a large, wide open area outside, and will use as many of the buildings and open spaces that your space can accommodate. This program can work in a large hall, but it may get a bit squishy and very noisy at times. In terms of group size, anything from 10 to 15 people works best.

The list of zany activities you could use at each activity station is endless. To get you started, adapt the following previously described activities (listed in no particular order) to run over 10 to 15 minutes with a small group.

Paper Plane Contest
Finger-Snaps
Leaning Tower of Feetza
Human Machines
Circle the Circle
Signature Bingo
Mintie Game
Stick Around
Top Monkey
Celebrity Head

Themes are always useful to connect activities. I have used an international theme successfully many times; for example, you could frame Leaning Tower of Feetza as hailing from Italy, and Celebrity Head as saluting America.

You will need a facilitator to brief and lead each of the activities – they can either stay with the same team, and present each of the different activities in sequence, or simply stick to one station, and present the same activity to all of the teams as they rotate through. Use a loud siren, whistle or other device to indicate when you would like the teams to rotate to the next activity. If you have spread the activities over a wide geographical area, supply each team with a map to assist them to locate the next activity in the sequence.

If you sense that your groups would be more motivated if there was a 'competition' of sorts, then go ahead and devise a scheme that will award points for completion of each activity.

Variations

- Using a slightly international theme, here are four more exercises you could try.

  - **Olympic Torch Relay.** With a balloon perched between his or her knees, a person will straddle to an object positioned about 20 metres (60') away and return to their team as quickly as possible without losing their balloon. He or she will then pass the balloon to the next team member (without using hands) to repeat the process until everyone has straddled.

  - **French Necking.** Ask your group to form a straight line. The person at the front of the line places an orange (or other similarly round object) between their chin and their neck, and passes it to his or her neighbour without using their limbs. The orange is passed from neck to neck down to the end of the line, and then in reverse back to the start of the line.

  - **Aussie Lifesaver Pass.** Your group forms a straight line, and each person holds a toothpick in their mouth. The person at the front of the line places one 'lifesaver' lolly (or other small candy with a hole in it) onto their toothpick. Without using hands or limbs, the group's goal is to pass as many lifesavers down the line to the last person as possible within the specified time frame.

  - **Inner Tube Relay.** Standing about 20 metres (65') away from an object, one person from a team places a large inner tube around their waist, in addition to other accoutrements such as a hat, scarf and flippers. On "GO," this person quickly races around the said object and returns to their team. At which point, he or she de-robes to allow the next person to repeat the process until everyone has run.

BLUESTAROPOLY

Think 'giant board game' that occupies a lot of people simultaneously

AT A GLANCE

Several teams roll a dice simultaneously to rotate a path around a giant
board game and accomplish a series of
random, zany activities as they progress.

WHAT YOU NEED

Giant (paper) game board
Various props, as determined by your
activities
Several big dice
1 – 2 hours

WHAT TO DO

I developed this idea whilst working
as a Camp Leader at Blue Star Camps,
North Carolina for five years. For several of those years, my mission was to
mix and occupy approximately 200 staff
for an hour or so, all at the same time,
as part of the 'evening entertainment.'
Alllllllright.

Your first job is to list a ton of zany
activities and tasks for a number of
small groups, or teams to accomplish.
It's not an exhaustive list, but check out

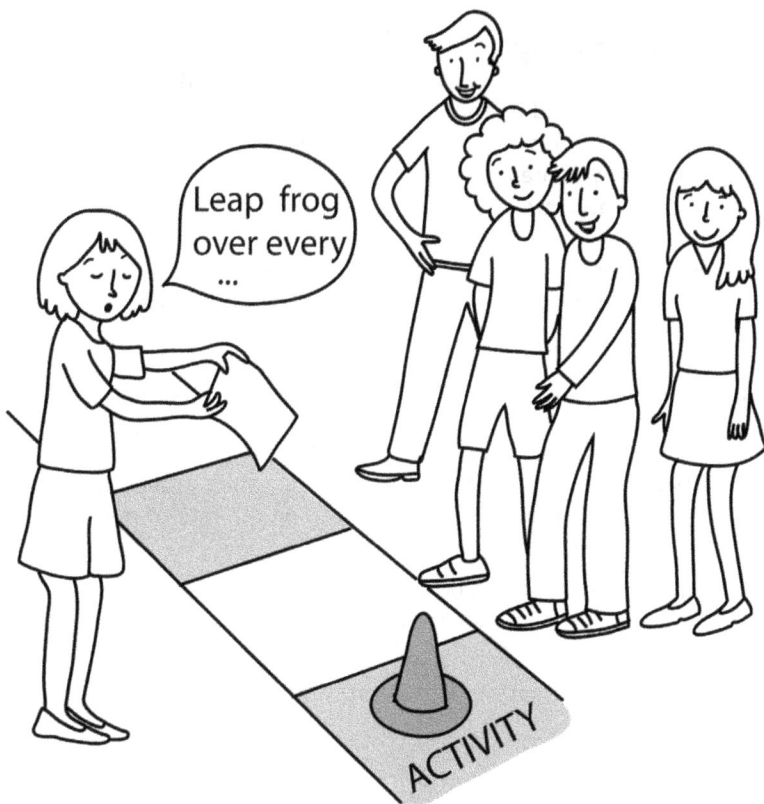

the ideas on page 239 to get you rolling.

Next, you want to build the biggest game board you have ever seen, complete with squares that run around the perimeter much like a Monopoly board. I used strips of roll-paper, taped together and then painted on the squares. Inside each square, I painted a large number, and on every third or fourth square I painted the word "ACTIVITY." Thinking back, I reckon the Board had close to 60 squares, and there were about 20 that had "ACTIVITY" written on them.

For added effect, I also painted a number of square cardboard boxes to look like huge dice. Regular playing dice work fine, of course, but I figured that if everything else was going to be as large as life, the dice should be too.

Once you have these two arduous tasks out of the way, you are ready to go. Separate your group into a number of teams, 10 to 15 people each. Lay out the Board and ask each group to sit in a spot around the outside of it. Place a few dice around the perimeter of the Board, and distribute a list of activities to each 'leader' (perhaps your colleagues) who will supervise a particular team.

Before starting, ask each team to offer some object that can be used to identify their position on the Board, e.g., a hat or shoe. Unlike most board games, do not start every team from the same point – spread the starting points evenly around the Board.

On "GO," each team rolls the dice, and moves their object the corresponding number of spaces forward onto a new square (there's no waiting for turns). Every time a team lands on an "ACTIVITY" square, their leader will consult the list and announce the next activity. Upon accomplishing the exercise, a team is entitled to roll the dice again.

Each team continues to rotate around the Board until they have completed every activity on their list. Or, they retire because they're knackered! I have never seen this activity fail to deliver extraordinary results.

Variations

- Assign the numbers on the squares of the Board to correspond to a number on the Activity List. In this case, each team will rotate around the Board a prescribed number of times, and depending on the fate of their dice, may or may not participate in the full list of exercises.

- Add squares that reward and penalise teams as they land on them. For example, "MOVE TWO SQUARES BACK," or "TAKE A LOLLY FROM THE JAR."

MASTERMIND RELAY

An assortment of 'out-of-the-box' problem-solving exercises

AT A GLANCE

Individuals or teams are challenged to accomplish as many creative, out-of-the-box thinking problems as they can within a set time frame.

WHAT YOU NEED

Set of printed 'Mastermind' activities
Set of 'Mastermind' props (optional)
Paper and pen for each team
1 - 2 hours

WHAT TO DO

I love this exercise because it is only limited by one's imagination. It's easy to set up, allows people to work at their own pace, and can occupy a group for a long time.

'Mastermind' activities, or 'brain-teasers' as they are sometimes called, require some form of focus, creativity and mental stimulation to be solved, and there are tons of them out there. You know the type – you need to think 'outside-of-the-box.' Here's an example: Why are the numbers listed below in the 'correct' sequence?

8   5   4   9   1   7   6   3   2   0

Some people will see the solution immediately, while others seem to get frustrated easily. Yet, with a little patience and some willing teamwork, many people quickly learn that they often short-change their problem-solving abilities.

There are two common presentation formats. If you have a large space to work in, you may choose to post a series of Mastermind problems at various stations throughout the area, and then ask your group to randomly move between each station. This is my favourite. Or, you may print off an identical set of Mastermind problems for each team, and invite them to work on the problems at a table. Either way, your first task is to develop a set of ten or more 'brain-teasing' problems.

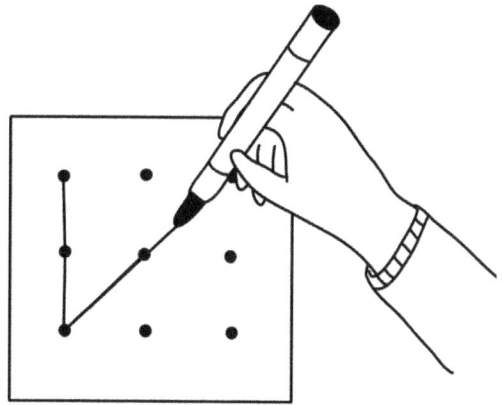

A range of problems I have often used with groups – which only require pen and paper to solve – are described on pages 240 to 241. For your convenience, some of these problems have been presented elsewhere in this book.

Once you have chosen your set of Mastermind problems, print them off. Then divide your group into teams of roughly ten people and explain that each team's goal is to solve as many of the problems as they can within a set time frame. Normally 45 to 60 minutes is sufficient, allowing time at the end to present the solutions and process any salient points.

By the way, the numbers are listed in alphabetical order.

Variations

- Integrate a series of 'prop' style problems too. For example, "USING A FULL DECK OF CARDS, BUILD THE TALLEST HOUSE OF CARDS," "HOW MANY JELLY-BEANS ARE INSIDE THIS JAR?" and "MAKING ONLY THREE ATTEMPTS, DROP A COIN INTO A CUP THAT IS RESTING AT THE BOTTOM OF A BUCKET OF WATER."
- Instruct your teams to move in a particular sequence around the Mastermind stations, allowing about five to ten minutes for each problem to be solved.

THE GREAT EGG DROP

A purposeful problem-solving team activity that comes with a thrilling climax

AT A GLANCE

Groups are provided with identical resources to build a 'vehicle' for an egg to travel from a tall height to the ground, hoping that it will prevent the egg from breaking upon impact.

WHAT YOU NEED

One egg (not hard-boiled) per team
20 plastic straws per team
1 metre (3-4') of masking tape per team
Paper and pens (optional)
A large plastic sheet
1 -2 hours

WHAT TO DO

Like many group activities, you are encouraged to really ham the presentation of this exercise to the max! Develop whatever scenario you care to think of, but be committed and make it fun.

For example, introduce yourself as a famous astro-physicist, and explain that you are seeking the best way for humans to land onto the surface of Mars. You plan to divide your group into competing teams of engineers, who will be charged with the responsi-

bility of building a space-craft that will not only transport humans safely to Mars, but more importantly, help them land in one piece. Whatever...you are now ready to present the task.

Each 'team' will be given identical resources – an egg, a set of straws, and a short strip of masking tape. The challenge is to build the strongest vehicle for an egg to safely travel a distance of 3 metres (10'). Why? Because, this is a prototype of the very spacecraft that will carry humans to Mars, of course! However, the distance will be gravity-fed, i.e., it will be dropped from a height, and land with a thud on the ground (that's why you need the plastic sheet – it's a landing platform).

Announce that each team's vehicle will be judged on engineering quality, efficiency of resource use, aesthetics, and naturally, on the survival of the egg. Feel free to add other forms of criteria too. Once all of the questions have been answered, and you have distributed the materials, declare that their time has begun. Allow at least 45 minutes for each team to prepare their craft.

Finally, the program reaches a huge

climax when each team returns and, under a veil of secrecy, submits their vehicle for testing. Leading with shouts of "10, 9, 8, 7..." and so on, you drop each vehicle from a height – one at a time (standing on a table works pretty well) – and await the results.

Typically, the egg will erupt with a fit of yellow and white splatter. Even a tiny flow of yolk will be sufficient for the crowd to go wild. Sunny-side up, anyone?

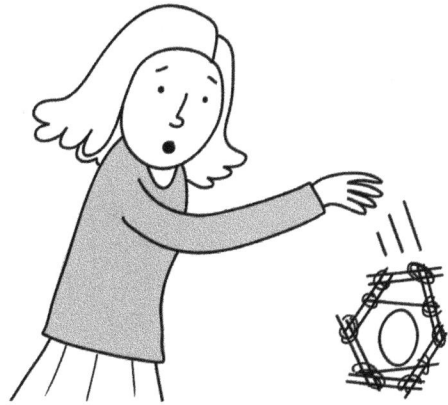

Variations

- Add a variety of materials to those above, such as balloons, rubber bands, cotton wool, etc.

- Ask each group, as part of their overall objective, to prepare a short presentation to accompany the launch of their 'vehicle.' Paper and pens can be used to design a 'marketing campaign.' Points are further awarded for creativity, originality and believability of their spiel.

TEAM SCRABBLE

Just like the real thing, only bigger and played in teams

AT A GLANCE

Teams work together to form words on a giant SCRABBLE Board and aim to earn the most number of points for using as many of their letters as possible.

WHAT YOU NEED

Giant 'Scrabble' board
A set of alphabet cards
1 – 2 hours

WHAT TO DO

Another wonderful adaptation of a popular board game.

Your first task is to create a giant

SCRABBLE board. The real game board has 225 squares (15 rows x 15 columns), but feel free to make it as large as you wish. I have used strips of roll-paper taped together and painted with squares to produce a giant SCRABBLE board in the past, but most recently, I learned to use an OHP transparency, projected onto a wall or whiteboard. In this latter case, you either write the letters directly onto the whiteboard or the transparency (upon which you 'give-up' the corresponding letters in your pile).

Next, write the letters of the alphabet onto a set of index cards. As a guide,

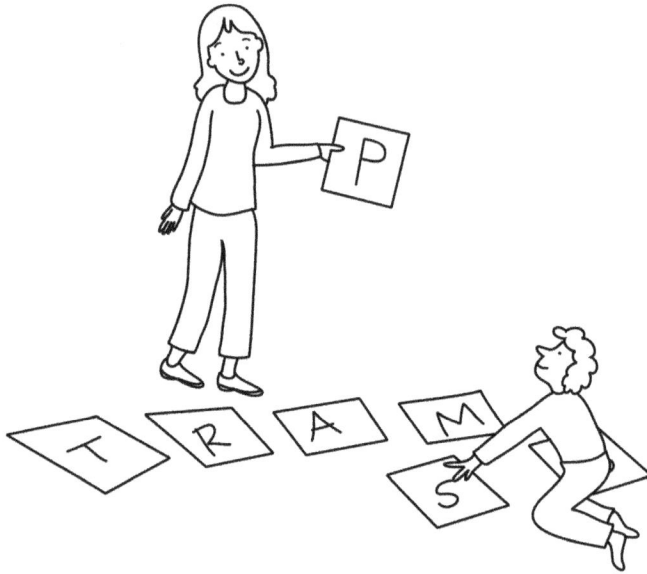

go to page 236 to view how many of what letters are used in the traditional SCRABBLE game.

Upon dividing your group into several teams, the standard rules of SCRABBLE pretty much apply. Each team starts with seven letters and, in turn, places as many of these letters onto the Board to make a word. After the first word is formed, every succeeding word branches off all existing words. Teams replenish their letters from the 'extras pile' for every letter they just played to form a word. Proper names and places are not permitted, nor are acronyms and abbreviations. But, you set the rules as you see fit. Game continues until one team uses all of their letters (and there are none remaining in the extras pile).

The combined cognitive energy of several people teamed together to form a word is enormously rewarding. Feel free to score as you would in SCRABBLE by applying certain point values to each letter, and adding particular bonus squares, such as 'DOUBLE WORD SCORE.' Or, simply award points for every letter used and / or word formed.

Variations

- Place a symbol on certain squares throughout the Board which if 'played' (i.e., a letter lays atop of it), requires the group to complete a certain task or challenge. The team earns the score of their word provided they accomplish the task. See page 239 for a number of zany task ideas.

- Design a very large Board, and provide every team with an identical set of alphabet letters. One team is randomly chosen to place the first word, after which, any team in any order can form a new word (branching off all other existing words as per normal). The team to use all of their letters first wins.

FAMILY FEUD

Adapting a popular TV favourite to a large group setting

AT A GLANCE
Teams compete to guess the most popular responses to a series of 'survey' questions.

WHAT YOU NEED
Set of survey questions
Flip-chart paper or whiteboard
1 hour

WHAT TO DO
As a teen, my mother and I would watch Family Feud on the telly every week night religiously. I guess a lot of people did, but I doubt many of them also recorded the questions and answers to all those surveys. Well, ummm… I did. You're right, this is way geeky, but now it's a treasure trove of programming gold.

For those unfamiliar with the TV show, Family Feud pitted one family against another by asking them to guess the most common responses to a series of survey questions. For example, "WHEN DO PEOPLE CLOSE THEIR EYES?," and upon surveying 100 people, the top five answers were recorded as Sleep, Kiss, Sneeze, Think and Wash your Face. The challenge was to guess what these top responses were.

So, unless you also recorded the results of every Family Feud episode in a cheap exercise book during the late 1970s, your first step is to develop your own set of survey questions. It's simple, but it does take a little time and effort. To view a series of survey questions that I have had success with, look at page 243.

On a sheet of paper, write 10 to 20 questions, providing a space for a quick response, and ask as many people as you can (at least 50 to 100) to complete the survey – try your work colleagues, your classroom, your residential campers, etc. The key is to ask people to write the first thing that pops into their head – there is no 'right' answer. If it takes them longer than three minutes to complete the survey, they are thinking too hard. You then tabulate the results, take the top or most common four to six responses, and you are good to go.

Divide your group into small teams of say five to ten people, and ask one representative from each team to come forward. Next, explain that you will soon ask a survey question, and the first two people to respond (raise a hand, hit a buzzer, say their name, etc) will be invited to give their responses. Asking the quickest person first, whoever suggests the highest ranked response (according to the actual survey results) will be invited to have his or her team guess all of the remaining responses.

For example, if the two quickest people record the second and third ranked responses to the survey question, the team that offered the second ranked response will earn the right to guess all of the other responses, i.e., the top, fourth, fifth, etc ranked responses. Record all correct responses on flip-chart paper or a whiteboard as they are guessed.

If this team correctly guesses all responses, they win the round.

However, if they fail to guess the full set of survey responses, the team that earlier gave the second quickest response gets a go. If this team can guess at least one of the missing responses, they win the round. But, if they also fail to guess at least one of the remaining responses, then every other team is entitled to put forward one guess. Award points to every team that contributes a response that matches any of the missing answers.

Please note, even though in the beginning only one team gets to guess all of the survey responses, all other teams still need to be engaged in the process because they may be asked at any time to contribute a response, if the teams before them fail to earn the points. A brilliant mechanism to keep people involved.

Invite a new person from each team to take the initial Family Feud challenge as each new survey question is announced. Propose ten or more survey questions to determine a 'winner.'

Variation

Propose a survey question to every team simultaneously, inviting each team to work together for two minutes to guess all of the survey responses. The team that has the most correct top ranked responses wins the points.

NAME THAT TUNE

In this quiz, earning the right to 'hit the buzzer' is as much fun as naming the tune

AT A GLANCE

Teams compete as they attempt to be first to perform a series of tasks and thereby, earn the right to guess the name of a musical tune that has just been played to the group.

WHAT YOU NEED

Tape / CD player
Recording of short musical snippets
2 packets of water crackers
Jar of peanut butter
A tray per team
Inner tube and pair of flippers per team (optional)
1 hour

WHAT TO DO

Your first big step is to prepare a tape or CD of short musical tunes. Record a lot of snippets (let's say, each plays for 1 to 15 seconds) from one or more musical genres that your group would have enjoyed over the years. So, if you're working with kids, be sure to record the beginning, chorus or other recognisable clips of current Top 40 songs and various hits from the past couple of years. Having said that, you always want to throw in a few obscure ones too. Use a range of genres, just lean heavily towards the dominant culture of your group. Remember, it's not a test – it's meant to be fun.

Now, gather your group, divide them into teams of say six to ten people, and ask them to sit along one wall or side of your playing space. Then, opposite each team, place a tray with several water crackers on which you have spread ample peanut butter.

Here's what happens. You announce to your group that you will soon play a short snippet of a song, and the goal for each group is to correctly guess the name and / or artist of the song. This part is often the easiest, but it's the 'earning the right' to hit the buzzer, so to speak, that is the hard part. Explain that upon identifying the tune, each team will designate one of its members to run to the place that is opposite of where they are seated, eat the peanut-butter smeared water cracker(s), and attempt to whistle as soon as possible. The first member of a team who can whistle properly (it's hard to do with peanut butter stuck to the roof of your mouth), is entitled to name that tune. If they are correct, their team earns a point, otherwise, the second-whistler-in-line may respond, and so on.

Word of caution: if you are one of the folks assigned to listen for the whistle, stand back! You are likely to be struck with fast-moving peanut-butter encrusted water cracker pieces in the process. And, yes there is a big difference between whistling and exhaling air at velocity.

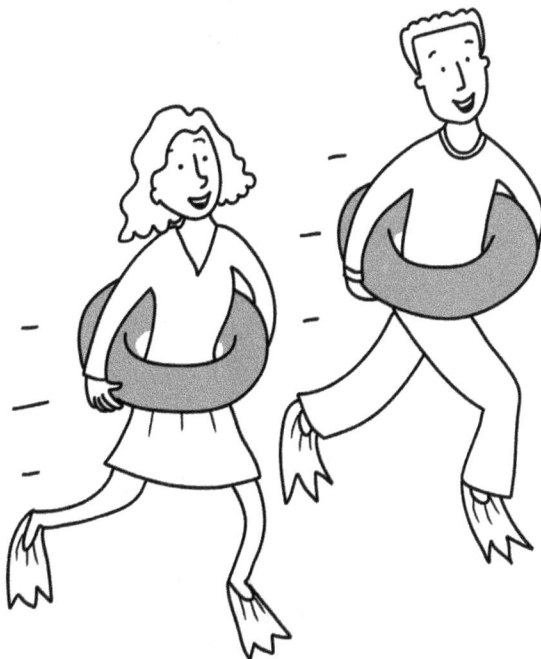

Encourage teams to send out a new person each time to run the 'peanut-butter-water-cracker-whistling' gauntlet. To really amp up the fun, place a large inner tube and a pair of flippers in front of each team. The member designated to go next, must put on the flippers and wear the inner tube around his or her waist while running to the tray. Either way, it's clearly more about having fun than it is about the music.

Variations

- Adapt this format to any 'quiz.' For example, ask a series of trivia questions, and invite a member from each team to perform 'a task' before earning the right to answer.

- Record a series of everyday sounds and noises as the 'tunes.'

- Rather than songs, record a series of TV show and / or movie themes as the 'tunes.'

SCAVENGER HUNT

A treasure hunt with a twist – nothing is hidden, but you still have to find things

AT A GLANCE

Teams are challenged to find as many items on a list of peculiar 'objects' to earn a varying number of points, within a set time limit.

WHAT YOU NEED

List of obscure objects or 'things' that need to be found

1 hour

WHAT TO DO

Upon dividing your group into teams of about 8 to 12 people, issue a list of objects that they need to find, and let them go. Yep, apart from developing your list of 'objects' in advance, that's it.

I recommend that the list ranges from the simple (a magazine) to the unlikely (a 1970 coin) to the bizarre (an emu feather). It's a good idea to have a wide selection of objects, because you'll always be amazed at what people can discover and / or get their hands on.

Here's a sample list that will give you a few ideas to start with:

Red hat
Fifty dollar note
Foreign currency
Dictionary
Yellow flower
Telephone book from another city
Photo of Princess Diana
Chicken breast bone (wish bone)
A tooth
Longest leaf
Glass Coca-Cola bottle
Monogrammed handkerchief

Naturally, you need to compile a list of objects that will not only be fun to collect, but will in some cases be

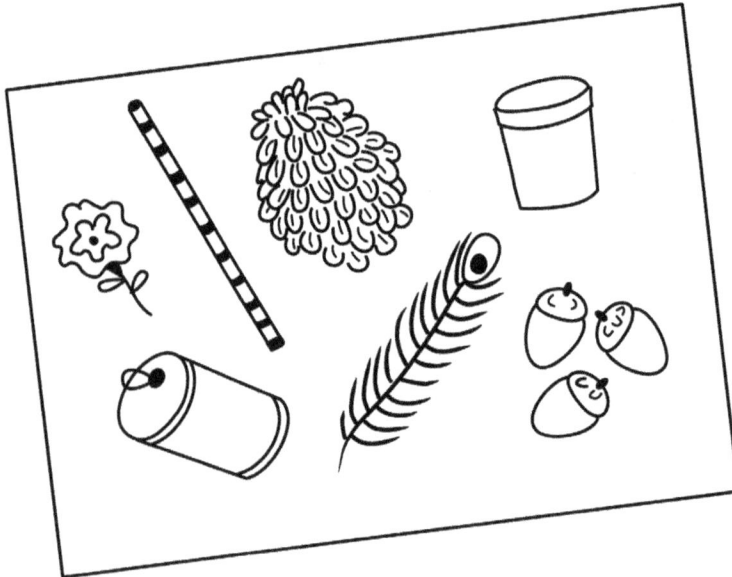

difficult to find. Challenge is, after all, the essence of this form of treasure hunt. Allow as long as you like for the scavenge to endure, but anything up to an hour is normally plenty of time. Award one point per item, or give certain harder-to-find items extra bonus points.

Variations

- Develop a list of ridiculous things, such as an 'A P B J,' 'snail egg,' 'tweed,' 'zipper zapper,' etc, and see what your groups come up with. Very inventive, and a wonderful game to inspire creativity.
- Compile a list of 'things' that have a common theme, such as nautical, animal, clothing, horticultural, etc.
- Look at Treasure Hunt below for a description of another 'hunt' variation.

TREASURE HUNT

Excellent team-based activity that can cover a lot of ground

AT A GLANCE

Teams search high and low within a defined area to 'find' as many unusual items of value as they can within a specified time period.

WHAT YOU NEED

List of 'treasures' that need to be located or hidden

A map marking the boundaries of the search area

A compass for each team (optional)

1 – 2 hours

WHAT TO DO

Your first task is to locate or hide a variety of 'treasured items' in and around a defined area for your group to uncover. Note, that to 'locate' is intended to mean that your group will simply note an item's appearance, whereas an object that has been hidden must be found, collected and carried back to the start. Either way, the hunt often requires a lot of preparation, and then, upon locating or hiding the items, you will need to develop a series of clues that will guide the teams to their position. The clues can be as obvious as "LOOK UNDER A BIG RED ROCK," to the more cryptic-style clues which will take some working out. Cryptic clues are more fun, but will take a lot more effort to develop.

Armed with a list of clues or 'treasures' to find, there are two ways you may choose to move your group – once they have been separated into teams – about the area:

- Sporadically, where the teams can discover the treasures in whatever order they choose; or
- Sequentially, where you issue a set of instructions with navigational hints (like compass bearings) to

guide the teams in a particular sequence to the locale of each treasure.

In this latter case, you may consider starting each team in a different spot (in the navigational sequence) to prevent 'follow-the-leader' tactics. Either way, ensure that the boundaries are really clear to everyone before they set off on their treks.

Scoring can be as simple as awarding one point per item found, or endowing certain harder-to-find items with more points than easier-to-find items. The team with the most points wins.

Variations

- Issue a digital camera to each team, and ask them to record the 'treasure' on film, so to speak, to prove that they found it.

- Rather than collect items, navigate the teams around a set course to answer a variety of questions along the way. For example, a treasure located in a natural bushland setting could ask "WHAT IS THE NAME OF THE RED FLOWER LOCATED AT THE BASE OF THE BURNT TRUNK?." Or, questions developed in a more urban environment may ask "WHAT TIME DOES THE PHARMACY OPEN ON SUNDAYS?" because the team passes the Pharmacy as part of the course. The most correct answers wins.

- For a hunt that actually brings home the treasure, see Scavenger Hunt on the previous page.

CITY SEARCH

Adventurous wide game that can tap into the creative energies of your group

AT A GLANCE

Teams are challenged to trek across a wide area in their quest for 'answers,' recording their adventures on film as they go. They are then to prepare a short creative presentation (involving their photographs) about their journey.

WHAT YOU NEED

List of quests or questions that need to be 'solved' for each team

A digital camera for each team (optional)

Small amount of cash (optional)

1 - 3 hours

WHAT TO DO

Owing to the truly adventurous nature of this exercise, it will not suit every group. You'll see why in a moment.

While some preparation is necessary for this activity, most of the energy and creativity comes from your group as the various teams work together to search for an answer or answers along their journey. At a minimum, you will need to prepare a list of one or more quests or questions for the groups to solve during their journey.

The key to this activity is in the framing of it. You need to give your group a reason to be wandering out and about their neighbourhood and / or country-side. So, with some gusto, you could announce that their mission is as significant as the search for the meaning of life, or as simple as conducting a survey about the merits of cleaning your teeth. Make it fun, make it crazy, but provide plenty of scope for the groups to be creative within the chosen framework.

To be a little more specific, provide each group with a number of quests or questions that they have to solve along their journey. Examples could include finding the 'upside-down' building, the details of a tombstone older than 1800, the tastiest pastries, someone named 'Elsie' or a person who can speak three languages.

In any case, this activity is all about adventure – neither you nor your group should know what to expect from their travels. And, herein lies the beauty (and inherent risk) of this activity. Given lots of room to move, the various teams you send out on their 'search' are encouraged to be as creative as possible. And, using their collective skills and ideally, a digital camera to record the events of their journey, combine their energies and newly-gained knowledge to perform a little show for the rest of the group to enjoy at the end.

The (optional) cash is a useful stipend to cover incidental expenses such as snacks and public transport for each team, if you anticipate the search to be long and spread over a wide area.

This activity works best if you can provide up to half a day in your program to allow the groups to undertake their journey, review their photographs and then prepare for their performances.

You can dispense with the photography and still achieve a rewarding outcome, but the truth of viewing snapshots of the actual journey is an exciting feature often woven into many group performances with spectacular effect.

Variations

- Develop a unique set of questions for each team to ponder along their journey, to cover a lot more material in the presentations.

- The questions could also reflect a particular theme, such as a topic you are wishing to study, for example architecture, community living, or urban humour.

ACTIVITY SUPPLEMENTS

This section is designed to unclutter the main body of the text with the solutions, lists and activity templates that I refer to in certain activity descriptions. If you need more ideas, or help, drop me an email at **mark@markcollard.com**

Nonsense Numbers
Acronyms
Wordles
Alphabet Equations
Alphabet Cards (Four Letter Word)
Minute Mysteries
Charade Line
In The Manner Of The Word
Zany Activities & Tasks
Mastermind Relay
Mastermind Relay Solutions
Family Feud

NONSENSE NUMBERS (PAGE 53)

CATEGORY	GUIDELINES	BONUS POINTS
Birthdays	1 pt for each different month	5 pts for holidays, leap year, born on same day
Birthplace	1 pt for each different state	5 pts for outside of this country
Pedestrian	Points for each different shoe size - Total all sizes.	5 pts for size 12 or larger, or size 5 or smaller
Travel	1 pt for visit to each site: Eiffel Tower, Empire State Building Sydney Harbour Bridge, London Bali, The Pyramids	5 pts for Mecca, Taj Mahal or Antarctica or any African nation
Celebrity	1 pt for each appearance on / in: TV, radio, newspaper / magazine (must be mentioned by name)	5 pts for all three media
Adventures	1 pt for rock-climbing, abseiling, scuba diving, horseback riding, whitewater rafting	5 pts for bungee jumping, skydiving, climbing 10,000+ foot mountain peak
Siblings	1 pt for each sibling (includes adopted, step, half-sibling)	5 pts for multiple births
Voyager	1 pt for each continent visited	10 pts for all seven continents
Surnames	1 pt for each letter of the alphabet	5 pts for each non-English character / letter
Linguistics	1 pt for each language fluency	5 pts for 3 or more languages
Longevity	1 pt for each year between the oldest and youngest member	5 pts for each decade represented, e.g.,0-10 yrs, teens, 20s, 30s, etc.

Group Identity Quotient (sum of all category scores) _____

ACRONYM ANSWERS (PAGE 57)

PIN	Personal Identification Number
DOA	Dead On Arrival
QANTAS	Queensland and Northern Territory Aerial Service
LASER	Light Amplification by Stimulated Emission of Radiation
NATO	North Atlantic Treaty Organisation
AD	Anno Domini
ANZAC	Australian and New Zealand Army Corp
FAQ	Frequently Asked Questions
BBC	British Broadcasting Commission
BMW	Bavarian Motor Works
LED	Light Emitting Diode
HMS	Her (His) Majesty's Ship
RAM	Random Access Memory
FUBAR	Fouled Up Beyond All Recognition
NIMBY	Not In My Back Yard
ATM	Automatic Teller Machine
SCUBA	Self Contained Underwater Breathing Apparatus
pH	Potential of Hydrogen
MGM	Metro-Goldwyn Mayer
WHO	World Health Organisation
FUNN	Functional Understanding Not Necessary
UFO	Unidentified Flying Object
DINK	Double Income No Kids
RSVP	Répondez S'il Vous Plaît
MASH	Mobile Army Surgical Hospital
GSOH	Good Sense of Humour
CEO	Chief Executive Officer
UNESCO	United Nations Educational, Scientific & Cultural Organisation
ISBN	International Standard Book Number
IVF	In-Vitro Fertilisation

WORDLE ANSWERS (PAGE 59)

This is just a very small sample of Wordles that I have come across over the years. If you are looking for more, take a look at Silver Bullets, by Karl Rohnke, or enter "WORDLES" into any decent internet search engine and prepare to be bamboozled.
The answers appear at the end of the table.

OHOLENE	SNOW WIND RAIN FEELING	BLOU**C**SE	HOROBOD
EVER EVER EVER EVER EVER	M E A L	R O ROADS D S	AM**U**OUS
OWHER	STEP PETS PETS	VAD ERS	B A E D U M R
B B B B A A A A R R R R G G G G	PLACE 3:46PM	LIB + LIB	ZERO TV
DICTATORSHIP LIVING	WEAR LONG	GEG GGE GGE GEG	R|E|A|D|I|N|G
GOEOD K MOAOD W	GIVE GET GIVE GET GIVE GET GIVE GET	J U YOU S ME T	SIGHT LOVE SIGHT SIGHT SIGHT
ping WILLOW	DENIM AWL AWL	BEND SDRAW	DEATH LIFE

DEAL	1 2 3 4 ^{5} 6 7	PLAY PLAY PLAY PLAY	MUM **MUM**
PARK PARK	*C C C C*	MONEY = $\sqrt{EVIL}$	HOPPIN
DICTNRY	B OW	PARD ME	YOURSELF LOOK
BUSINES	B O B	INILT	↓ END
_____ DRIVE	PAR TWO	MILL1ON	POLMUMICE
DNA 4TH	LUC KY	T RN	d D d D W D d D d

Hole In One

Feeling Under The Weather

See-Through Blouse

Robin Hood

For Ever and Ever

Square Meal

Cross Roads

Ambiguous

Middle of Nowhere

One Step Forward, Two Steps Back

Space Invaders

Bermuda Triangle

Up For Grabs

Right Place, Right Time

Adlib

Nothing on TV

Living under a Dictatorship

Long Underwear

Scrambled Eggs

Reading Between the Lines

Wake Up In a Good Mood

Forgive and Forget

Just Between You and Me
Love at First Sight
Weeping Willow
Denim Overalls
Bend Over Backwards
Life After Death
Big Deal
High Five
Foreplay
Minimum and Maximum
Parallel Park
High Seas
Money Is the Root Of All Evil
Shopping Centre
Abridged Dictionary

Elbow
Pardon Me
Look After Yourself
Start Of Business
Bob Up and Down
Nothing In It
Beginning of The End
Line Drive
Par Under Two
One In a Million
Mother in Law
Back and Forth
Lucky Break
No U-Turn
Wind In All Directions

ALPHABET EQUATIONS (PAGE 60)

26 = L of the A	Letters of the Alphabet
7 = W of the AW	Wonders of the Ancient World
1001 = AN	Arabian Nights
12 = S of the Z	Stars of the Zodiac
54 = C in a P with Js	Cards in a Pack with Jokers
88 = PK	Piano Keys
13 = S on the AF	Stripes on the American Flag
32 = DF at which WF	Degrees Fahrenheit at which Water Freezes
18 = H on a GC	Holes on a Golf Course
57 = HV	Heinz Varieties
66 = B in the B	Books in the Bible
50 = S in the U	States in the Union
14 = D in a F	Days in a Fortnight
21 = D on a D	Dots on a Dice
3 = S and you're O	Strikes and you're Out
6 = S on a H	Sides on a Hexagon
4 = Q in a G	Quarts in a Gallon
90 = D in a RA	Degrees in a Right Angle
29 = D in F in a LY	Days in February in a Leap Year
64 = S on a CB	Squares on a Chess Board

ALPHABET CARDS (PAGE 222)

The following number of alphabet letters is modelled on the tiles of the English SCRABBLE game. There are one hundred letters in total.

A x 9   B x 2   C x 2   D x 4   E x 12   F x 2   G x 3   H x 2   I x 9   J x 1

K x 1   L x 4   M x 2   N x 6   O x 8   P x 2   Q x 1   R x 6   S x 4   T x 6

U x 4   V x 2   W x 2   X x 1   Y x 2   Z x 1   Blank x 2

Can every letter of the alphabet be used once only to form a SCRABBLE puzzle of words? Yes. There are many ways to do it, but here's just one in case you or any of your groups suggest that it can't be done.

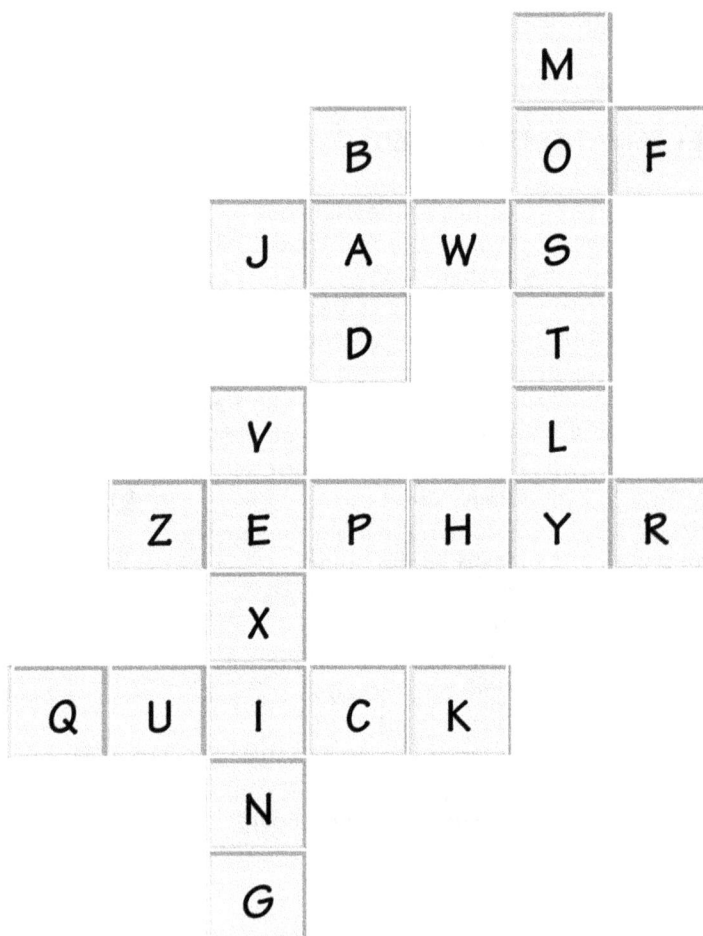

```
                              M
              B               O   F
          J   A   W   S
              D               T
          V                   L
      Z   E   P   H   Y   R
          X
      Q   U   I   C   K
          N
          G
```

MINUTE MYSTERIES (PAGE 193)

- **Facts:** Romeo and Juliet are dead, lying in a puddle of water with broken glass everywhere. How did they die?

  Solution: Romeo and Juliet were fish, and their fish tank fell and crashed to the floor.

- **Facts:** A man pushes his car in front of a hotel, and declares bankruptcy. Why?

  Solution: The man is playing Monopoly and cannot afford to pay the 'rent.'

- **Facts:** Two men go into a bar and order exactly the same drink. The first man chugs his drink while the second man savours it. Within an hour, the second man dies. Why?

  Solution: The ice cubes in both drinks were poisoned. The first man did not give time for the ice to melt. The second man sipped his drink, so the ice had time to release its poison.

- **Facts:** A man leaves home, and when he returns to it a short while later, he finds two men in masks waiting for him. Why?

  Solution: The man is a baseball player, and the two men in masks are the umpire and catcher.

- **Facts:** Fifty people were sitting in a cabin eating a snack when they suddenly died. What happened?

  Solution: The people were sitting in an airplane cabin, and the plane crashed killing everyone on board.

- **Facts:** A man lives on the 40th floor of an apartment building. Everyday, the man rides the elevator to the Ground floor and goes to work. Yet, when the man returns home, he gets off at the 10th floor, and then walks 30 flights of stairs up to his apartment. Why?

  Solution: The man is very short and can only reach the button of the 10th floor.

- **Facts:** A man is found dead lying in the middle of a field with a pack on his back. What happened?

  Solution: The man is a skydiver and his parachute failed.

- **Facts:** A father and son are involved in a car accident. The father dies, but the boy survives and is taken to the hospital for surgery. A grey-haired, bespectacled surgeon looks at the boy and says, "I cannot operate on this boy - he's my son." Why?

  Solution: The surgeon is the boy's mother.

- **Facts:** A man wearing a scuba suit is found dead in the middle of a forest. What happened?

  Solution: The man was diving in a nearby lake when he was accidentally scooped up by a water bomber to dump a load of water on a bush fire.

- **Facts:** A man walks into a bar and asks for a drink. The barman pulls out a gun. The man says "Thank you" and leaves. What happened?

  Solution: The man had hiccups, but the gun scares them away.

CHARADE LINE (PAGE 199)

Here are a few of my favourite 'sure-fire' Charade Line stories to get your started. There's no limit to the number of stories you could invent. Indeed, ask a volunteer from your group to offer a story.

Story One

You walk in swinging a bag in your hand. You stop and pull out a chair and a fishing rod from the bag. You sit down, throw your line into the river, and start to relax. Suddenly, your fishing line starts to tug, and you feverishly try to reel it in. After much effort, you are disappointed to discover an old rubber boot hanging off the end of your line. You empty the water out of the boot, put it on your foot, and walk off.

Story Two

You pull an elephant into your 'space' on a long rope. You tie the rope at a stake, and then dip a rag in a bucket and start to wash the side of the elephant jumping high to get all the way to the top. You crawl underneath, wash the elephant's belly and legs. You also go to the front and wash the trunk inside and out and wash the elephant's ears as well.

Story Three

You are a high school beauty pageant contestant, anxiously awaiting the announcement of the winner. Suddenly you hear your name! You now step forward to receive your crown and roses. Then as you take your victory walk down the aisle, waving to the crowd, you encounter many misfortunes. First, you are allergic to the roses, so you begin to sneeze, but you keep on going waving and sneezing to the crowd. Then, on the way back up the aisle, your high heel breaks and you finish the walk with one heel missing!

Story Four

You're are a pregnant bird about to give birth flying around the room. As you fly, you are gathering materials for your nest. You pick up many items, varying in size, shape and weight. Once you make your nest, you lay your egg. The egg miraculously hatches, so you quickly leave the nest to pull a worm from the ground, and return to feed it to your baby.

IN THE MANNER OF THE WORD (PAGE 203)

Here's a list of fun adverbs to try with your group:

SLOWLY	CLOSELY	QUICKLY	EAGERLY	NERVOUSLY
CAREFULLY	ANGRILY	HAPPILY	BLANKLY	CONSCIENTIOUSLY
HEROICALLY	IMPATIENTLY	LOVINGLY	NIMBLY	PRECISELY
QUIETLY	STIFFLY	THANKFULLY	SMUGLY	SOFTLY

ZANY ACTIVITIES & TASKS

The list of activities which follow are ideal for Be Prepared (page 213), BlueStarOpoly (page 217) and any other crazy tabloid-sports team-based game you can think of.

If you're looking to mix it up with a few passive, brain-teaser kinds of ideas, take a peek at Wordles (page 59), Acronyms (page 57), Alphabet Equations (page 60) and Mastermind Relay (page 219).

- Standing next to each other, form a straight line, and perform 'The Wave' up and down the line three times.

- Shake the hands of at least three people in a neighbouring group.

- Everyone whistle a full verse of "When the Saints Come Marching In."

- Spend three minutes to create a team cheer. Wait to be called upon to present it to the other groups.

- Standing up, form the word B E A C H with your bodies.

- Carefully jump on the back of another person in your group, and be piggy-backed around the perimeter of the room / hall / playing space and return to your spot.

- Inflate a balloon and have everyone in your group touch the balloon, without touching anyone else in the group.

- Build the tallest free-standing structure you can in two minutes using only your shoes / footwear.

- Sing and perform the full Hokey Pokey song and dance for two different parts of your anatomy, e.g., "You put your left foot in..."

- Pick a partner in your group and waltz with them for 15 seconds.

- Involving everyone, perform one complete line of leap frog.

- Everyone lies down on their backs, with arms and legs in the air, wiggles and yells out, "DEAD ANT, DEAD ANT, DEAD ANT..."

- In classic operatic style, everyone sing, "Twinkle Twinkle Little Star."

- Spend one minute to form the most bizarre 'group sculpture' in which every group member must be physically touching another person, but no more than two feet can be touching the floor (other parts of your anatomy can touch the floor, however).

- While sitting down, form a circle holding hands. Now, stand up as a group while not letting go of your partner's hands.

- Take five minutes to share and determine who has the best, funniest, yet cleanest joke in your group, and nominate them to tell the joke in front of all other groups.

- Sing one verse of [enter name of your National Anthem].

- Everyone approach [enter name of leader or other key person] and shake their hand.

- Nominate one person to speak spontaneously for 60 seconds non-stop about bananas.

- Name five movies that are currently showing at your local cinema.

- Everyone swaps a piece of outer-clothing with someone in the group and wears it.

- Everyone stands, joins hands and rotates clockwise two times, stops and then rotates two times in the other direction.

- Everyone gets down on their hands and knees and barks like a dog.

- From a seated position, everyone stands up, claps three times, and then sits down.

MASTERMIND RELAY (PAGE 219)

The following list offers a variety of wonderful 'Mastermind Relay' problems that require only a pen and paper to present and / or solve. The solutions are on page 242.

1. Wordles – take your pick from page 59.

2. Alphabet Equations – take your pick from page 60.

3. The two lines of letters below are distinctly different. Identify one of the possible next letters in the sequence of each line:

   A   X   I   M   E   __

   B   Q   D   J   U   __

4. Drawing only three lines, divide this circle into eight sections.

5. How many squares are there in the figure below?

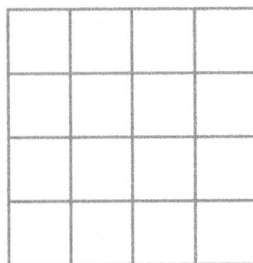

6. How many triangles are there in the figure below?

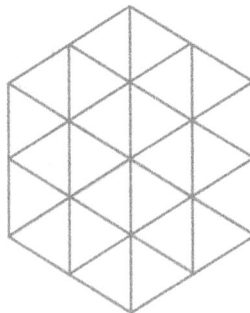

7. Connect all nine dots below by drawing only four straight consecutive lines. That is, once you begin drawing, you are not permitted to lift your pen off the paper.

11. What is a one syllable word that becomes a three syllable word when you add just one letter?

12. A rooster is sitting on top of a pitched roof. If the rooster lays an egg, on which side of the roof will it fall?

13. Together a bow and arrow cost $21.00. On its own, the bow costs $20.00 more than the arrow. How much does the arrow cost?

14. There is a house on a mountain. All four walls face south. A bear passes by. What colour is the bear?

15. You have eight identical-looking balls. Every ball weighs the same, except one ball is slightly heavier. Using a set of scales only twice (you know, as in the Libran zodiac sign), describe how can you identify which ball is heavier. Note, it is not possible to discern the weight difference by holding the balls in your hand.

8. You have only two buckets. One holds exactly 3 litres, and the other holds exactly 5 litres. Other than an unlimited supply of water from a tap, there are no other props or materials available to assist you to solve this problem. Your task: Using only the two containers, describe how you can measure exactly 4 litres of water. Your solution should aim to solve the problem using the least amount of water.

9. Draw only two squares so that each of the nine dots below is in a separate space, i.e., no two dots will be inside a set of four lines.

10. What can you find twice in a week, once in a year, but never in a day?

MASTERMIND RELAY SOLUTIONS

1. Wordle solutions can be found on page 233.

2. Alphabet Equations solutions can be found on page 235.

3. The letters in the top line are made exclusively of straight lines, whereas the letters in the bottom line are made of at least one curved line. Letters that can be added to the top line include E, F, I, L, M, N, V, W, X and Y. Letters which can be added to the bottom line are: B, D, O, P, Q and S.

4.

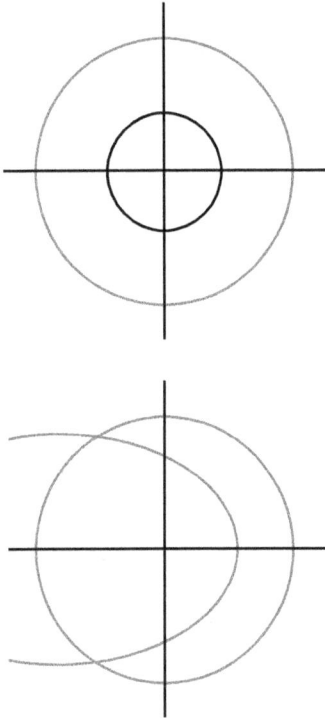

5. Thirty

6. Thirty-eight

7.

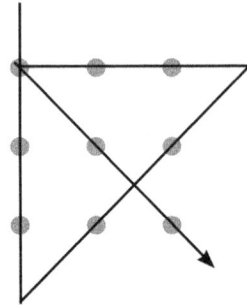

8. Fill the 3 litre bucket and pour contents into the 5 litre bucket. Refill the 3 litre bucket, and pour 2 litres into the 5 litre bucket (to fill it). Empty 5 litre bucket. Pour remaining 1 litre of water from 3 litre bucket into 5 litre bucket. Refill 3 litre bucket and empty all contents into 5 litre bucket to supply it with exactly 4 litres of water. Total amount of water used is 3 + 3 + 3 = 9 litres.

9.

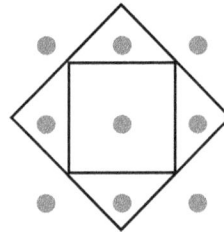

10. The letter E

11. Add A to ARE and get AREA

12. Neither, as roosters do not lay eggs

13. 50 cents

14. White, it is a polar bear (the house is situated on the North Pole).

15. Place three balls on each side of the scales. If they are balanced, then the next use of the scales with the two remaining balls will determine the heavier ball. However, if one set of three balls is heavier, remove all balls, and place any two of these "heavier" three balls on the scales (one each side). If these two are balanced, then the one that has not been weighed is the heavier ball. Otherwise, the heavier of the two balls is it.

FAMILY FEUD (PAGE 223)

I have not provided the top survey responses to these questions (after all, they are at least 25 years old), but they are good survey starting points.

- Name a type of place where the seats are uncomfortable.
- Name something that takes a lot of chewing.
- Name an article of clothing that gets in the way.
- Name something that you shake.
- Name an occupation that is over-paid.
- Name something that can fall from the sky.
- Name something people do but do not like doing.
- Name something you can fill.
- Name something that people wear that is false.
- Name something associated with a bunny.
- Name a famous giant.
- Name a type of food that starts with the letter 'P.'
- Name a small creature that terrifies people.
- Name something that people squeeze.
- Name something that has wrinkles.
- Name something that has horns.
- Besides a house, name a place where people live.
- Name something that buzzes.
- Name a food that often burns.
- Name something that is clear.

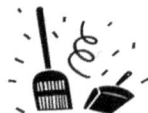

CLEANING UP

This section is designed to give you a few pointers about the many resources that Project Adventure can provide to help you get the most out of your programs.

There are literally dozens of training workshops, books and resources out there designed to enhance the knowledge and activities you have gleaned from this publication. But, to be honest, the best way to learn this stuff is to do it. Get out there, have some fun, fail forwards and remain inventive. By attending one of our training workshops, you will not only get to see many of the activities described in this book played out for real, but also discover many invaluable networking opportunities.

Project Adventure's primary mission is to help people use Adventure as a catalyst for personal and professional change and growth. Feel free to contact us at any time if you would like support as you introduce Adventure into your setting. We've been doing it for more than 36 years, and in almost every possible setting imaginable. Bring the Adventure home, and have fun!

PROGRAMMING PHILOSOPHIES

The discussion that follows aims to provide you – whether you are new or not-so-new to the programming field – with a few guiding philosophies designed to inspire successful programming.

The success of your program relies on many factors, and most of them are profoundly related to preparation. Your training as a program provider, the breadth and depth of your repertoire of activities, even the arrangement of logistics such as equipment, food, venue and transport (where necessary) are all important to your success. Yet, I would argue that the most critical factor to success is the preparation of your group.

The programming philosophies of Sequencing, Challenge by Choice, FUNN, the Full Value Contract and the Experiential Learning Cycle, are intended to support and promote the attributes of success in your program – risk-taking, fun, challenge and safety (both emotional and physical). In other words, they are designed to invite your group to play, trust and learn.

These four philosophies inspire all of the activities in this book, indeed, pretty much all of Project Adventure's curricula. Work hard to keep them in focus and in play at all times.

SEQUENCING

The Right Activity at the Right Time

While there is no magic formula that can help achieve the perfect program, often a critical ingredient to achieving success is the sequence of your program's activities.

Sequencing involves making the order of your activities appropriate to the needs of your group. This means preparing your group, mentally, physically and emotionally, for what's coming up. Did you get that? Preparation; sequencing is all about preparing your group for the challenges that lie ahead so that it may be successful (whatever that means). This is a not a new concept, but one that applies across the board regardless of content.

The use of 'lead-up' activities is crucial. Without appropriate lead-up, you may jump into activities for which your group is not ready. For example, the use of a few introductory or 'ice-breaker' activities, that help people get to know one another and allow them to 'let off some steam,' may assist you to create a more exciting and energetic start to your program. Or perhaps, these activities could highlight a particular learning outcome or skill that you will want to call on later.

Sequencing also relates to the necessary adjustments that are made to your program as you progress – activity by activity. Because all activities elicit a range of behaviours, feelings and attitudes – and no two groups are the same – your own observations of what is going on with a specific group is an equally important key to sequencing.

For example, the fact that you've played 'Gotcha' a dozen times, and most groups you work with exhibit similar characteristics, does not mean that each group should not be treated individually. It also means that even though the agenda says that your group is supposed to be doing a certain activity at a certain time, if your group members are not ready, don't push them. Change what you had originally planned to do, or get to it after you've added a few more preparatory activities.

It's like 'learning to crawl before you walk.' Appropriate sequencing will lead your group to success, but it will also help you to create a fun, positive experience in which everyone feels valued, rather than pushed.

Here's a simple model of sequencing that I've found useful over the years.

Ice-breakers
Activities that provide opportunities for your group to 'get to know one another,' have fun and begin to feel more comfortable with each other. Initially, you can expect this stage of the program to be success-oriented, with an emphasis on fun, high interaction and minimal decision-making.

De-inhibitizers
Now that people are feeling more comfortable with each other, you and the program, invite them to engage in activities that assume more risks – emotional, physical and mental – to extend their comfort zone. The emphasis is on trying (rather than success / failure), having fun and creating a positive atmosphere in which the group can begin to feel supported and more confident.

Skill Development
At this stage, your group possesses the requisite skills (and preparedness) to communicate, cooperate and trust one another within a safe, supportive environment. They are now prepared for the 'main event.'. This can range from developing skills in a basketball clinic, to developing social skills within the framework of a series of problem-solving activities, to creating a sense of play / performance for a high-energy, fun evening program to conclude a three-day school camp.

Ask yourself, "What skills am I trying to develop within this group and / or program?" i.e., is it fun, recreation, social skills, sporting prowess, etc. Then, think about how you can best prepare your group to meet this challenge, and importantly, achieve success.

Where Are the 'Trust' Activities?

When I first started out, I believed that 'trust' activities were a necessary, yet separate stage of this sequencing model, i.e., after de-inhibitizers but before the big development stuff. But, I find that this view just doesn't fit anymore.

As my understanding of programming has developed, I have realised that trust was something I fostered right from the time I said, "Hi, my name is Mark." Sure, there are specific trust exercises (like the Fall from Height activity, aka Trust Fall) that are devoted to the development of trust, and owing to their nature, are properly conducted later rather than sooner in a program's sequence. But the earliest signs of trust are born in the cacophony of laughter and smiles you generate in your first lead-up activities, maybe even in your introduction.

Trust is gradually developed as your sequence of activities progresses. It begins slowly, and builds so that by the time you are about to embark on more challenging parts of your program – probably the very reason they are together, to develop a particular set of skills perchance – you have the necessary levels of trust in place to achieve a successful (i.e., desired) outcome.

If it helps, imagine that when your group first forms, or just arrives at your venue, etc, it is possible to enumerate the level of trust, and let's say it's zero. Not good, not bad, just nothing there. Clearly, your objective as a prudent facilitator would be to guide your group through your program, ever–nudging the trust levels higher and higher. That is to say, you're aiming to move the trust of the group from a zero to something positive.

Of course, many groups exist with elements of trust already established, which is great – they'll start with something positive just waiting to be

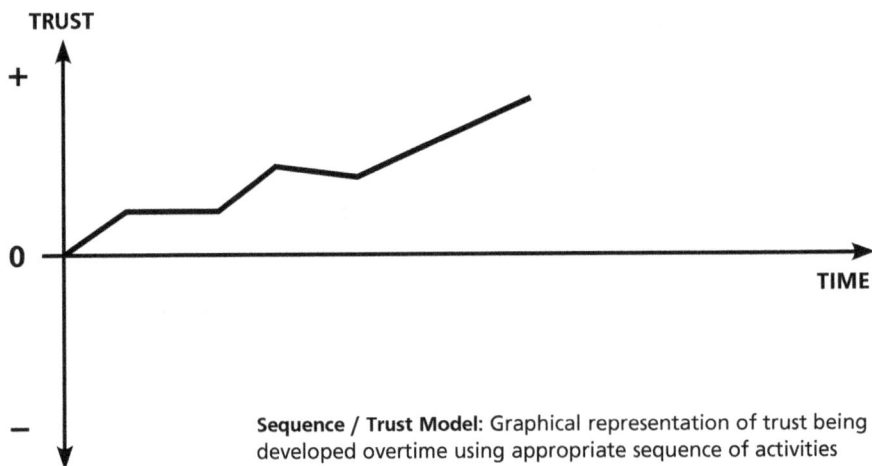

Sequence / Trust Model: Graphical representation of trust being developed overtime using appropriate sequence of activities

developed further. But sadly, the reality for some groups is a measure of trust that is lower then zero! In these circumstances, the best result we could hope to achieve would be to lift a negative to a zero.

Do you get my drift? No matter where the trust starts, the more it develops, the more your group will play, share and learn. And, that's all we ever want, isn't it?

So, this raises a question – how do you measure trust anyway?

You can't, you kinda just get a feel for things, a sense of the 'I-feel safe' factor, so to speak. And that's why it is so important to constantly observe the interactions and reactions of your group, and make necessary adjustments (to the way you say things and plan and present activities) as you go. And like most things, the more you deliver, the better you get at judging the fluctuating levels of trust, needs and skills of your group.

Choosing the Right Activity

There are a number of tools 'out there' that aim to assist you in assessing a group's needs at any given time. I can think of no better instrument than GRABBSS. Regard it as your 'grab-bag' of clues that can help you juggle the plethora of activities you have in mind and determine which one is 'right' for now.

GRABBSS is a series of questions divided across seven key modalities, that is, elements you can observe and evaluate about your group, and the impact your program is having on its development. One element is not necessarily more important than another, but the acronym reads as follows:

Goals How does this activity relate to the goals of the group and overall program, or those that you see emerging? Basically, this element is asking, why are you doing the activity?

Readiness Is the group ready (mentally, emotionally, physically) to do the activity? What needs to change before the group has the ability to undertake the next stage of the program?

Affect What is the feeling of the group? What sensations are they experiencing – boredom, excitement, apathy, resistance, etc?

Behaviour How are the group or individuals acting? Are the interactions between members positive or negative for the group? How cooperative are they? Will their behaviour be appropriate for the activity?

Body What are the physical abilities of the group? What physical characteristics of the group will impact the program? Are the individuals tired, do they substance abuse, do any individuals have a disability, are they hot or cold, etc?

Stage What stage of development is the group in? Using Bruce Tuckman's popular rhyming schema to describe the varying levels, are they Forming, Storming, Norming, Performing or Transforming? Does the group need additional skills to function at a higher level (stage) of development? Generally speaking, the higher the level of group development, the more challenging your activities can be.

Setting What is the physical setting of the program, and the 'cultural' background of the participants? Are you inside or outside, secluded or likely to be disturbed? Is the space limited? How long have the people known / worked with each other?

In essence, you are constantly asking yourself these types of questions to help you make an informed decision about what is appropriate for the 'what's next?,' i.e., what does my group need next?

For example, you may be working with a school group for the purposes of developing team and communication skills. Even though your agenda suggests that you should do X activity at Y time, if the group has not demonstrated that it has the skills necessary to succeed (i.e., the group is not ready), then you are well advised to alter your program sequence. Add one or more alternative activities that match the skills of the group and aim to develop their readiness for the desired activity.

Or, perhaps the group is ready to move onto the next more challenging activity, but 'cooled' down significantly during the debrief – throw in a quick 'warm-up' to move their bodies once again before proceeding.

Now, it would be nice if for every answer you came up with for each of the elements of GRABBSS you could assign a number, and then just calculate the sum of all these numbers, and this was the pointer to what activity to use next. Yes, it would be nice, but totally implausible. Rather, GRABBSS is about observing your group and planning on the run – all of the time. It is a constant asking, what does my group need to achieve success?

For a more elaborate description of GRABBSS, check out *Exploring Islands of Healing* by Jim Schoel and Richard Maizell.

CHALLENGE BY CHOICE
Empowering through choice

This means you give the participants a realm of choice to determine their level of involvement (or challenge) in a given activity. Nobody is forced to do anything they don't want to do. The motivation to participate comes from within, rather than from external influences.

A choice to not participate in a particular activity, or (more often) to assume a role that is more comfortable for the participant, is always respected. Real success and learning occurs only when individuals choose and commit to their own standards and goals that are personally meaningful.

However, operating within the programmatic context of Challenge by Choice is more than simply allowing your participants to say, "No" and pull out of an activity. It's about creating a safe learning environment for your participants which invites them to make appropriate decisions in an atmosphere they expect will support them. In essence, you aim to empower them to make their own decisions, but also encourage them to 'give it a go.'

As a program facilitator, you have to be profoundly related to this concept of choice, especially in relation to your program design, and your language. It's one thing to say "…this program operates under the philosophy of Challenge by Choice…." But it's entirely another thing to be responsible for a program that speaks to, honours and fosters an atmosphere in which people genuinely feel comfortable to make decisions regarding the level of their participation.

Creating a 'safe' learning environment (in the physical, mental and emotional senses of the word) should be your primary concern. A program in which people feel safe to express themselves, and experience the freedom to make their own decisions will produce an extraordinary environment in which play, trust and learning can occur and flourish. Challenge by Choice is one of the most important tools you can employ to help you develop this atmosphere.

A Word on Participation

Many people – facilitators and participants alike – often confuse Challenge by Choice with 'participation.' This is a simple trap, but people can participate in so many different ways, it's more than just running around.

A case in point. I was involved in the delivery of a pilot program that integrated police recruits and, for the want of a better word, 'street kids.' To be honest, I would be hard-stretched to think of two more diametrically opposed groups. Anyway, our first morning was humming along, but two of the street kids chose not to join in. Challenge by Choice had been introduced, so I respected their decisions to sit out. However, I did take it personally, that even despite a full-on-fun program, my encouragement and the urging of their friends to join in (i.e., "it's really cool"), I could not motivate these two girls to participate. By day's end, the two girls did not move from their comfortable sidelined position. Sigh....

And then, it happened. To wrap up the day, the top brass of the police squadron asked the group a few questions, a debrief of sorts, including the old standard "...What did you learn about each other today?" To my shock, one of the two girls put up her hand. I'm thinking, "What entitles you to answer this question – you didn't participate all day?" She replied something to the effect of "I didn't think the coppers would laugh at the same things we did!" And then it hit me.

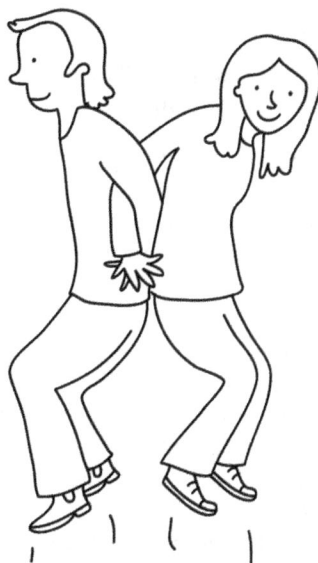

This girl had been participating all day, she just chose (for whatever reasons) to do it from the sidelines. It was one of those 'aha' moments we all strive for, and was only made possible because of the atmosphere that had been developed during the day, particularly enabled by the use of Challenge by Choice. If this girl had been forced to participate, I am certain the result would have been very different.

The choice not to do an activity can be just as powerful as the choice to do it – in all cases, the choice – if it is made freely and in an atmosphere of support – will empower the individual. When viewed in this context, Challenge by Choice becomes a challenge of choice.

FUNN

Fun Is Okay, Or People Learn If They Are Having Fun

Obvious fun is very hard to stand away from, and so the FUNN – a whimsical acronym for Functional Understanding Not Necessary – element of a program goes a long way toward involving everyone's participation. Karl Rohnke, author of many Project Adventure titles, coined this term, and it it's an absolute gem. Applied liberally throughout your program, it says "If it's fun, I want to be a part of it."

FUNN means that it's okay to be involved in an activity for no other purpose than to enjoy it. You, or your participants, do not need to have a special reason to do an activity. Do it for the laughs, the play and the good feelings it creates. You will be surprised by the results. We should take fun more seriously!

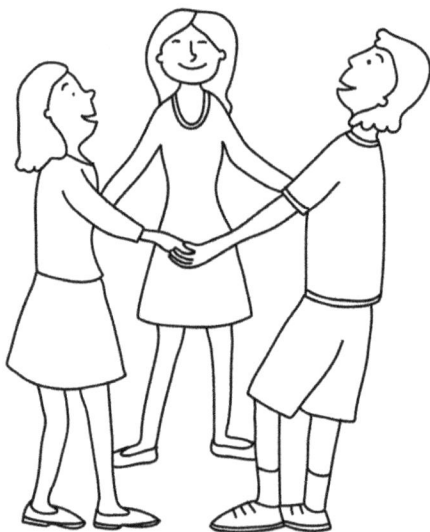

On the face of it, having fun during the course of a 'serious program' can appear to some people (dare I say, many decision makers) as folly; a serious waste of time and resources. Or, in other words, "Why are we playing childish games when we should be ... [feel free to add whatever serious intent you care to name here]?" This school of thought would have us believe that playing and learning is tantamount to throwing a bucket of dollar bills into the wind, and trying to catch as many of them as you can with oven mitts. You can't be serious, and I rejoin – that's exactly the point.

It is absolutely essential to inject a heavy dose of FUNN style activities into your program for, ironically, lots of valid, intrinsic reasons. I can not stress this enough. Programmatically, there are mondo motives for adding FUNN to your program – to invite people to laugh, to share, to play, loosen up, set the tone, or to change the pace, etc – all of which contribute manifestly to the development of trust. Full stop. Yes, FUNN is good, agreeable, contagious, its own reward, etc, etc. But it will also help facilitate your program goals – the beauty is, your participants don't need to understand that this is what's happening. It just goes on around them.

I often remark that "If in the midst of having an outrageous time today, you should stop and ask yourself 'Why are we doing this?,' then may I suggest you don't work too hard to find an answer – simply enjoy it for what it is." You see, I want the budding trust to sneak up on them. They'll see it as just having fun, but I know better. The old 'you-have-to-trust-each-other' while I wag my finger trick just doesn't work. Oh, and it's no fun either. Injecting FUNN into your program will give your participants the permission they crave to play – truly play – and happily for you, the motivation to generate a safe place, which inspires good sharing – which leads to trust – which can stimulate learning. Voila!

EXPERIENTIAL LEARNING CYCLE

Fun is often reason enough to use adventure-based activities. However, you can enhance the overall experience of your group if you take some time to reflect and talk about 'what just happened' in these activities. This time can help the program become a valuable and meaningful experience for everyone.

The Experiential Learning Cycle is the foundation of all experiential or Adventure-based programs. It proposes that the transfer of learning will be more effective if what is being learned is discovered though actual experience or, as it is sometimes referred to, 'learning by doing.'

However, simply engaging your group in a series of activities one after the other will not automatically effect learning. If your goal is to use a series of activities to enhance learning, you will need to facilitate the learning process – or in other words, process or debrief the experience.

Processing the Learning Experience

You may have heard the phrase "Let the mountains speak for themselves." It suggests that anything that your group may learn from an experience will happen of its own accord. Happily, this philosophy may work for those who heard the message. But what about those who didn't, or perhaps, heard the wrong message? They risk leaving your program without gaining any value from it, or worse, receiving a negative experience.

Clearly, the practice of simply 'doing' does not, in and of itself, create 'learning.' If your goal is to invite your group to have fun, then this 'hands-off' approach may be fine. But, if you are looking to have an impact on learning, you may need to 'facilitate' this process. Indeed, the process of reflecting upon an experience in order to gain meaning, and then connecting these meanings to 'real life' will provide many opportunities for learning. This process has been captured by David Kolb in four interrelated phases of what he refers to as the Experiential Learning Cycle.

This process (also referred to as a debrief, or review) provides an opportunity for members of your group to come forth with their own perceptions of 'what it all means.' Guided by your questions, participants can talk things out and tackle relevant issues, such as communication and leadership within the group. Within the context of a safe and supportive atmosphere, they can also provide feedback to one another and raise significant learning points.

Anecdotal evidence (i.e., lots of people tell me) suggests that many program leaders have difficulty with the processing or debriefing elements of an activity. We worry that we won't be good at it, or our group will resist talking about stuff, or put simply, the pressure of trawling for pearls of wisdom every time makes it all too hard. Well, relax. Volumes have been written about

The Experiential Learning Cycle

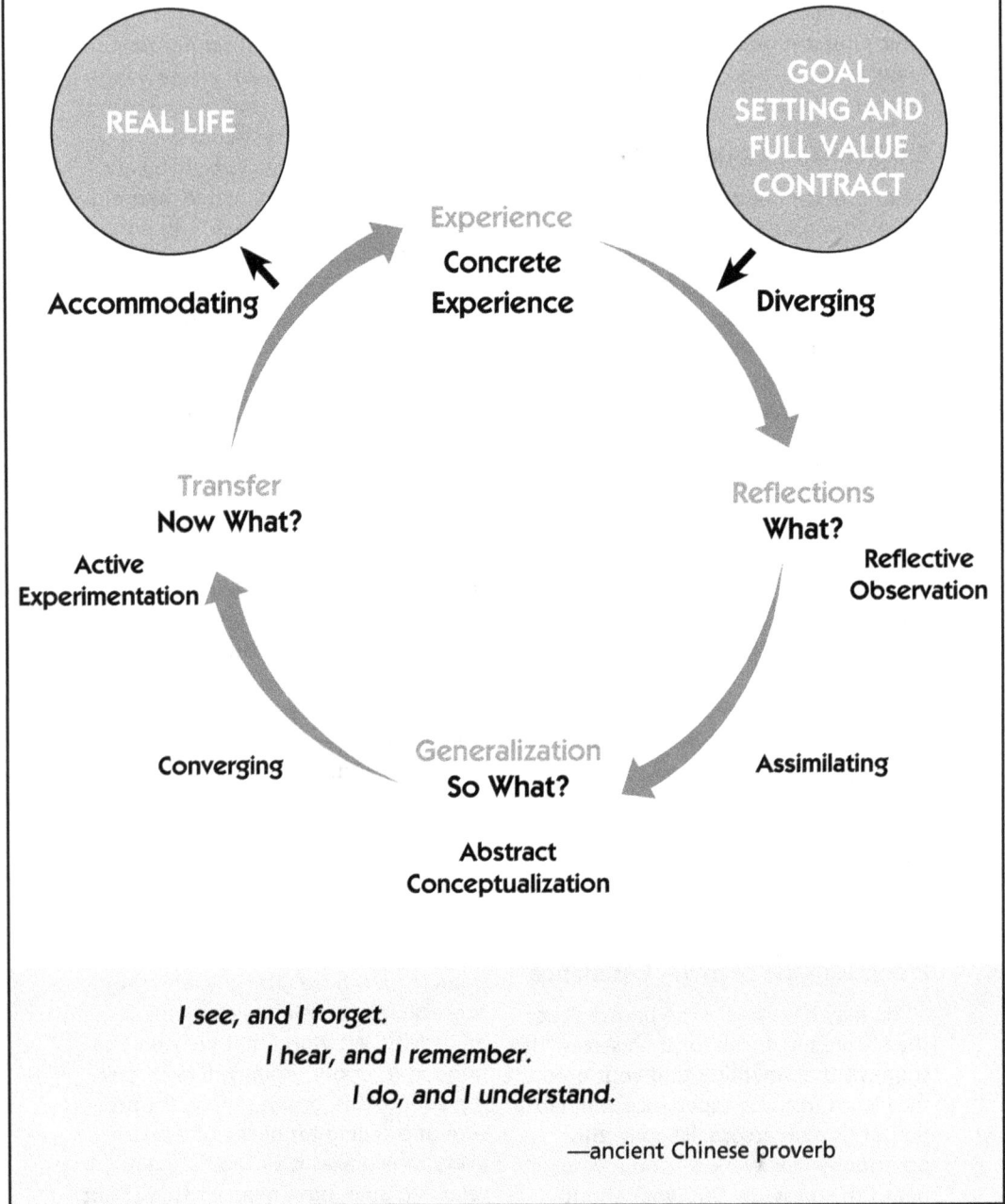

REAL LIFE

GOAL SETTING AND FULL VALUE CONTRACT

Accommodating

Experience
Concrete Experience

Diverging

Transfer
Now What?

Active Experimentation

Reflections
What?

Reflective Observation

Converging

Generalization
So What?

Assimilating

Abstract Conceptualization

I see, and I forget.

I hear, and I remember.

I do, and I understand.

—ancient Chinese proverb

the art and science of processing, and they pretty much all boil down to three simple steps.

What, So What, Now What?

Just as the activities in your program need to be sequenced carefully, you should also sequence your discussion.

1. **What?** Reflecting on the details of 'what happened' in the experience(s).

2. **So What?** Generalising these facts, making connections and looking for patterns.

3. **Now What?** Applying this information to the next activity, or ultimately, to people's real lives – at school, home, work and play.

Ease into your debrief by beginning with the facts. Ask 'What?' type questions to start with. This will get people talking, and to be honest, this is often the hardest part. Some examples may include, "What did the group do when the second beach ball was introduced?," "What methods were used by the group to solve the problem?" and "How did the group come to a decision?."

Then, if appropriate, you can move the discussion to the next step – interpreting or adding meaning to what happened. The 'So What?' step presupposes that we do something with what we hear, to find out what this all means, and perhaps make generalisations. "When groups are in discussion, it is best for one person to speak at a time" is a good example of a generalisation at work.

At this point it is important to ask questions that help the group find its own answers. This is a good place in which to address issues such as trust, communication, safety, leadership and cooperation. These 'So What?' type of questions may look like "What made the method of solving this problem so effective?," "Why did the group become frustrated?" or "How did it feel to be left out of the decision-making process?"

The most powerful step is moving the group on to consider the 'Now What?'. A standard question to ask is "What have we learned in this activity that we can apply to …. (whatever the reality is for this group)?." Sometimes, these connections are very clear, while other times the group has no idea. Again, this is where you come in.

Use questions that help your participants see the big picture, such as, "Give me an example of how we could improve our cooperation based on what we have learned from this activity" or "What will we do differently as a group next time?" and "What goals can we set for this group to improve your overall performance?."

Do not expect to see the blinding light every time you sit down with a group to discuss what's happened. But, if you are keen to draw more than a fun time out of your program, provide a structured reflection period from time to time. It will not only supply you with tons of valuable information about how your group is travelling, but will expand your group's learning opportunities.

FULL VALUE CONTRACT

Agreeing On How We Are Going To Look After Ourselves

Creating a safe, supportive and fun atmosphere has got to be one of the most important responsibilities of a program provider. To not focus on this

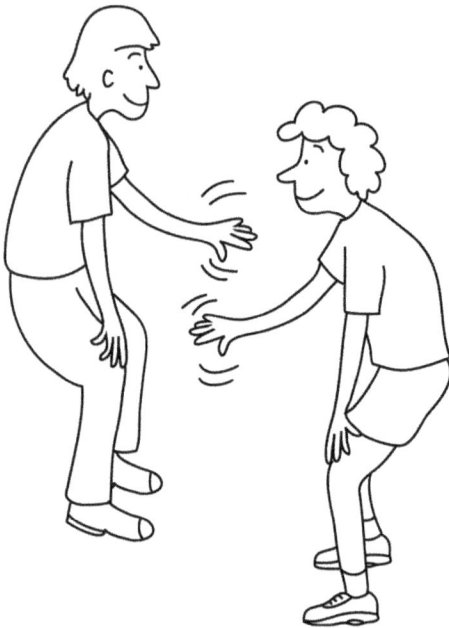

critical task, is akin to driving without a seat-belt – no matter how short or long the drive, there is always the chance of an accident.

The Full Value Contract is a bit like a seat-belt. It is an agreement (a device) that helps individuals and groups achieve their goals in a safe and supportive learning environment. No matter what group or program you care to mention – from your standard weekly two-hour basketball clinic to multi-day, residential Adventure programs – every one of them will benefit from the process of consciously defining what is expected of people's behaviours.

The Full Value Contract – in its many and varied forms – is the cornerstone of Project Adventure's work. With Full Value, you can establish workable group 'norms' (that is, accepted ways of being) that foster and manage appropriate behaviours. And it's always

'appropriate behaviours' for this group, right here, right now. Every group is necessarily different. In theory, you may expect values such as 'to be honest' or 'respect for every one' to be common across the board, but, in practice, the understanding of these concepts may vary widely.

What the 'Full Value Contract' Looks Like

Basically, the Full Value Contract or agreement is a statement (either written or oral) made by each member concerning their shared values and how they wish to be treated. Values such as respect, openness, acceptance of differences and patience are time-honoured contributions. 'No put-downs,' 'Alcohol- free,' 'Constructive feedback' and 'Everyone has an equal say' may be examples of more specific agreements for specific populations.

Importantly, the Full Value Contract ought to fit the unique goals, characteristics and spirit of your group. No matter what shape it may take, it is a shared creation, and should embrace three broad tasks:

1. To understand and create safe behavioural norms under which the group will operate;

2. Seek a commitment to adhere to these norms by everyone in the group; and

3. To accept a shared responsibility for the maintenance of the group.

Importantly, the inspiration for and the shape of whatever agreement is formed must reflect the needs and characteristics of your group and program design. The Full Value Contract you develop for a one-hour class with students will differ significantly from that created for a residential therapy group. So will the agreement formed between adjudicated youth and that developed for a one-day corporate training workshop.

Here are just three ideas regarding alternative designs:

Play Fair, Play Safe, Play Hard
Introduced 'as is' at the start of your program, perfect for short programs, and young people.

Be Here, Be Safe, Be Honest, Commit to Goals, Let Go & Move On, Care for Self & Others
Presented within a discussion of the six components, ideal for older youth and adults, and programs of a longer duration.

Do-It-Yourself
A creative means, by which you invite the group to come up with their own tenets of agreement – suitable for most ages. It may be written down (or drawn) or communicated verbally.

Keep in mind, and continuing the analogy of a seat-belt, consider the Full Value Contract as a fluid and continuous process. Sometimes, the seat belt may have to be really tight (for example, asking people to sign a written document that explicitly prescribes the agreement), or quite loose to allow some freedom of movement (where the group may alter the framework of the agreement as their skills develop).

Why Bother?

I can't tell you the number of times I have had a group explain to me that they don't need a 'full value thin-gee' because 'we all get along great.' These are the groups I worry about the most.

Of course, there are groups that really do care for one another, and echo a wonderfully safe and supportive environment in which to play and learn. But most groups, no matter the reason for their existence or length of program, will benefit from some form of shared, conscious agreement that governs their behaviour. Even groups that have been together for a long time – such as a school class, or a work-team – will gain a lot from the process of sharing and making conscious those aspects of their collective norms that are acceptable, and those that are not.

In my experience, much of the discussion reflects typically unwritten, unspoken laws of 'how we do things around here.' Naturally, for those groups that are just forming, there is no such thing.

Hence, even if the list of 'norms' is exactly the same for every member of the group, the process of actually sharing and making this agreement conscious is whole-heartedly beneficial.

Once it has been formed, a Full Value Contract presumes specific expectations for all group members, i.e., everyone knows where they stand. And then its full power may come to bear, because it transforms into a self-monitoring / policing agreement. Responsibility for the growth and safety of the group no longer rests solely with 'the leader.' If something is amiss, the Full Value Contract gives any individual permission to bring it to the attention of the group, and request that it be addressed.

Project Adventure Books and Publications

Project Adventure has been publishing books and materials for the field of Adventure Education since 1974. Our titles cover all aspects of Adventure – from games and initiatives to specific school-based curricula, from Challenge Ropes Course use to program safety, theory and practice.

Some of our most popular titles include:

Physical Education Curriculum – Elementary, Middle & High Schools by Jane Panicucci, with Alison Rheingold, Amy Kohut, Nancy Stratton and Lisa Faulkingham-Hunt

Achieving Fitness: An Adventure Activity Guide (Middle School to Adult) by Jane Panicucci with Lisa Faulkingham Hunt, Ila Sahai Prouty and Carolyn Masterson

Creating Healthy Habits: An Adventure Guide to Teaching Health and Wellness (Middle School) by Katie Kilty

Quick Silver by Karl Rohnke and Steve Butler

No Props: Great Games with No Equipment by Mark Collard

The Guide for Challenge Course Operations by Bob Ryan

Exploring Islands of Healing by Jim Schoel and Richard Maizell

Silver Bullets by Karl Rohnke

Cowstails & Cobras II by Karl Rohnke

Islands of Healing by Jim Schoel, Dick Prouty and Paul Radcliffe

Gold Nuggets: Readings for Experiential Education edited by Jim Schoel and Mike Stratton

Program Resources

Adventure programs, both with and without a Challenge Ropes Course, need accessories that can often be difficult to find or adapt. The Project Adventure resource catalogue provides an extensive range of innovative Adventure accessories – from fleeceballs to rubber chooks (chickens), floppy frisbees to boffers, from belay devices to challenge course hardware – to help you to administer your program.

For a complete listing of books, games and gear, visit our website www.pa.org

Training Workshops & Services

Public training workshops, conducted throughout the USA, Australia, Japan and New Zealand, aim to help you learn the skills to present safe and valuable adventure-based programs. Project Adventure also provides a wide range of services, including:

Challenge Ropes Course Design & Installation

Program Consultation

For a complete listing of workshop types and dates, visit our website www.pa.org

PA International Network

Project Adventure, Inc.
701 Cabot Street
Beverly MA 01915 – 1027 USA

Phone (978)-524-4500 or
(800)-468-8898
Fax (978)-524-4502 Web www.pa.org
Email info@pa.org

For more information on our licensed affiliates in Japan, New Zealand, Australia and Singapore, email international@pa.org or call (800)-468-8898.

Project Adventure has offices / partnerships in several southeast Asian, South American and European countries.

Contact Project Adventure at (800) 468-8898 or info@pa.org for current contact details.

About the Author

Mark Collard grew up in Melbourne Australia, the eldest of three children. He earned his Bachelor of Business (Accounting) degree, before heading to New York to study for his MBA – his eyes firmly set on the 'tie and collar' world.

Then, having led programs with youth groups and summer camps in both Australia and the United States for many years, Mark's eyes were properly opened in 1989 when he attended his first Project Adventure workshop led by Karl Rohnke. Things haven't been the same since.

Mark joined Project Adventure Australia in 1990, and was employed full-time by the organisation for ten years during which he was the principal manager, one of only two Certified Trainers in Australia, training coordinator, sometimes Challenge Course builder, and overall office dog's body.

Leaving PAA's full-time employ in 1999, Mark has continued to deliver many Adventure programs for the Project as a contract facilitator, particularly throughout Australia, the United States and Southeast Asia. In 2005, Project Adventure published Mark's first American title No Props: Great Games with No Equipment.

Beyond playing games and writing activity books, Mark keeps busy as a voice-over artist and Master of Ceremonies (think weddings, trivia programs, conferences, etc) and still dreams of hosting his own TV show. You can check his progress at www.markcollard.com

For the record, Mark has walked gingerly on a bed of nails, been lucky enough to find not one, but five four-leaf clovers, seen a moon-bow (a rainbow at night), and calculates that he has spent more than four months of his life trapped inside a steel tube (flying through the air at 800 km/h).

Mark lives in a mud-brick home in Melbourne's outer east with his most gorgeous wife Gilly, and counts his work with Project Adventure as some of the 'funnest' times of his life.

He would be really happy to hear from you at any time – email him at **mark@markcollard.com**

ACTIVITY INDEX

playmeo

Visit **playmeo.com/activities** to view 100s of fun group games & activities, many of which are featured in this book. Get step-by-step instructions, video tutorials, leadership tips & so much more.

www.ingramcontent.com/pod-product-compliance
Lightning Source LLC
Chambersburg PA
CBHW080246030426
42334CB00023BA/2723